Care of Drug Users in General Practice
a harm-minimisation approach

Edited by

Berry Beaumont
General Practitioner

Foreword by

William Clee
Chairman, Welsh Advisory Committee on
Drug and Alcohol Misuse

Radcliffe Medical Press

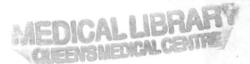

©1997 Berry Beaumont

Radcliffe Medical Press Ltd
18 Marcham Road, Abingdon, Oxon OX14 1AA, UK

Reprinted 1999

British Library Cataloguing in Publication Data

A catalogue record for this book is available from the British Library.

ISBN 1 85775 236 8

Library of Congress Cataloging-in-Publication Data is available.

Typeset by Advance Typesetting Ltd, Oxfordshire
Printed and bound by Biddles Ltd, Guildford and King's Lynn

Contents

1003391873

List of contributors

Clive Barrett
Clinical nurse specialist
Hurley Clinic
Ebenezer House
Kennington Lane
London, SE11 4HJ

Dr Berry Beaumont
General practitioner
The Surgery
2 Mitchison Road
London, N1 3NG

Dr Judy Bury
Primary Care Facilitator (HIV/AIDS and Drugs)
Spittal Street Centre
22–24 Spittal Street
Edinburgh, EH3 9DU

Julian Cohen
Consultant and trainer in drugs education
JDC Training and Consultancy
15 Church Street
Hadfield-via-Hyde
Cheshire, SK14 8AD

Dr Philip Fleming
Consultant psychiatrist
St James' Hospital
Locksway Road
Portsmouth
Hants, PO4 8LD

Dr Chris Ford
General practitioner
Brent and Harrow Substance Misuse Management Project
5 Jardine House
Harrovian Business Village
Bessborough Road
Harrow, HA1 3EX

Dr Clare Gerada
General practitioner
Hurley Clinic
Ebenezer House
Kennington Lane
London, SE11 4HJ

Dr Mary Hepburn
Senior Lecturer in women's reproductive health
Department of Obstetrics and Gynaecology, and of Social Policy and
    Social Work
Glasgow Royal Maternity Hospital
Rotten Row
Glasgow, G4 0NA

Dr Stefan Janikiewicz
General practitioner and Clinical Director for drugs and alcohol,
    Wirral and Chester
Moreton Health Clinic
8–10 Chadwick Street
Moreton
Wirral
Merseyside, L46 7XA

Dr Katie Kemp
General practitioner
Primary care unit
National Temperance Hospital
118 Hampstead Road
London, NW1 2LT

Dr Edwin Martin
General practitioner
2 Goldington Road
Bedford, MK40 3NL

Greg Poulter
Solicitor
Release
388 Old Street
London, EC1V 9LT

James Tighe
Team manager
Hurley Clinic
Ebenezer House
Kennington Lane
London, SE11 4HJ

Dr Tom Waller
General practitioner
Novocastria
Sandy Lane
Waldringfield
Woodbridge
Suffolk, IP12 4QY

Brian Whitehead
Counsellor in general practice
Lonsdale Medical Centre
24 Lonsdale Road
London, NW6 6RR

Foreword

I was delighted to accept when invited to contribute the Foreword to this important new publication. My own involvement with caring for drug users in general practice came about by chance. I had just taken-up a partnership as a full-time general practitioner in a large group practice in 1985, when I was confronted with an outbreak of hepatitis B among amphetamine injectors on a small council estate in the Welsh Valleys. Over the next 12 months, my partners and I dealt with 34 cases of hepatitis B and screened and counselled many more intravenous users.

Well before the publication of the influential ACMD report *AIDS and Drug Misuse, Part I* in 1988, we addressed this situation by practising, without realizing at the time, what are now commonly accepted harm minimization/harm reduction philosophies.

The problems which surfaced on uncovering this unexpectedly large group of intravenous drug users so suddenly proved to be legion and we quickly learned the most important strategy in dealing with this client group – joint working and shared care in a multi-disciplinary–multiagency setting.

Over the next year an invaluable trust-based relationship was established with the whole polydrug misusing sub-culture in our area. This has continued to form the basis of our extensive ongoing work in the primary care setting and our crucial ability to establish early contact with new users. I have firmly believed ever since that the GP is in an ideal and pivotal position to act as the initial point of contact with a drug user. A unique insight into family dynamics and background can only come from the in-depth knowledge held by a well-structured primary health care team who are best placed to co-ordinate close follow-up, supervision and support in the family/community setting, particularly when young children and pregnancies are involved. They can also liaise with secondary and other services, take a pro-active role in health promotional issues and aim to minimize or reduce the harm drug users may do to themselves, the family and the community in general.

Due to the lack of services for problem drug users from the statutory (both health and social services) and voluntary sectors in my own area at the time of the hepatitis B outbreak, I became involved, together with a health visitor, a social worker and a number of concerned mothers, in establishing what is now a thriving voluntary sector street agency, Taff Ely Drug Support (TEDS). My continuing involvement has taught me the vital role to be played by the voluntary sector in working with primary care and other agencies involved with the drug user. I feel that a strong case should now be made for increased resourcing of treatment and rehabilitation as being the most cost-effective way of achieving crime prevention and improved community safety from drug-related crime.

I was appointed in May 1996 by the Secretary of State for Wales to chair the new Welsh Advisory Committee on Drug and Alcohol Misuse. During the initial high level of media exposure, I clearly laid down my own areas of priority for the new Welsh Strategy which included:

- more emphasis on the involvement of primary care including the care of pregnant drug users

- services, structures and joint working strategies for dealing with young people

- the engaging of the community as a whole in dealing with the problem

- a new emphasis on prevention and education

- crisis intervention

- addressing the issues around hepatitis C

- tackling what I believe will become one of the most important areas of concern over the next few years – 'dual diagnosis'.

I also stressed the need to look in detail at issues concerning benzodiazepines and stimulant use in the whole polydrug use setting. All this work is underpinned by the multidisciplinary–multiagency joint working principle.

When given sight of the chapter layout of this book, I was delighted to see the common agenda that so clearly exists – no stone is left unturned. The list of contributors is impressive and the quality and content of the chapters outstanding.

Our experience in Wales with the 'substance misuse' approach, covering illicit drugs, prescription drugs, over-the-counter preparations, volatile substances and alcohol should prove an interesting testing ground for this concept over the next few years. It should also point the way forward for other areas in the UK, where many DATs are already starting to look at this broader approach.

I greatly welcome the publication of this book as a valuable new GP resource. It will act as a stimulus to encourage more primary care physicians to take a positive role in engaging this client group in a shared care environment.

William Clee
Chairman, Welsh Advisory Committee on Drug
and Alcohol Misuse
Member of Clinical Guidelines Working Group (DoH)
June 1997

Acknowledgements

I would like to thank all the people who have written chapters for this book, particularly Chris Ford whose additional contributions and support I have valued very much. Thanks must also go to the drug-using patients in my practice who have trusted me to provide their care. I have learnt a lot from listening to them. I am grateful to Brian Hurwitz for encouraging me to produce this book, and to Annie Beaumont and David Lawrence for their patience and support whilst it was being written.

Dr Berry Beaumont
June 1997

1

A GP's role: past, present and future

Tom Waller

Introduction

National strategy for the care of drug users in general practice has undergone profound change in recent years and is continuing to evolve. In less than 25 years, the treatment of opiate dependence has changed from maintenance prescribing to rigid abstinence-oriented treatment, back to a harm-minimization approach with a variety of substitution prescribing packages. In this time, general practitioners (GPs) have been variously expected to treat and not to treat patients with opiate dependence, and later exhorted to '… treat these patients and help them in every possible way'.[1] It is not surprising that this has led to confusion amongst GPs as to their role, and to controversy.

A clear understanding of the current approach, and the developments that have taken place leading up to it, may help GPs clarify their views as to the level of intervention that they are willing to give.

National strategy

National strategy is summarized in the 1995 White Paper *Tackling Drugs Together. A Strategy for England 1995–1998.*[2] There are similar strategies for Wales[3] and Scotland.[4] The strategy focuses on three areas:

- crime
- young people
- public health.

The following states the strategy purpose:

To take effective action by vigorous law enforcement, accessible treatment and a new emphasis on education and prevention to:

- increase the safety of communities from drug-related crime

- reduce the acceptability and availability of drugs to young people and

- reduce the health risks and other damage related to drug misuse.

National policy and GPs' management of drug misuse

With regard to the GP's role, the current approach is best summarized in the recommendations of the 1996 Task Force Report.[5] The Task Force was an independent body and had amongst its members a GP representative. It was set up by the government 'to conduct a comprehensive survey of clinical, operational and cost effectiveness of existing services for drug misusers' and to review current policy. It recommended the following.

- GPs have responsibility for the physical health needs of drug misusers within the provision of general medical services and should be encouraged to identify drug misuse, promote harm minimization, and where appropriate, refer to specialist services.

- The process of 'shared care', with appropriate support for GPs, should be available as widely as possible. Health authorities should encourage its expansion to enable GPs to take overall clinical responsibility for drug misusers and agree with a specialist a treatment plan that may involve the GP prescribing substitute opiate drugs.

- GPs should be sufficiently skilled to identify a problem drug misuser who may be consulting them for other, perhaps related, problems. This may require a programme of specialized training for some GPs.

- GPs should know to whom they can refer in a crisis and for ongoing support, either from specialist drug workers regularly attending their clinics, or by access to a named key worker in the local specialist agency.

- The service provided by the GP should be agreed with the Local Medical Committee and specialist services and should clearly set out the respective roles of the GP and the specialist services, and the support the GP can expect in delivering the service. Purchasers should ensure that GPs have straightforward access to urine-testing facilities.

- Where they have concerns about compliance with consumption arrangements, GPs should have access to facilities where supervised consumption can take place.

- The agreement between the Local Medical Committee and specialist services for the provision of shared care should include arrangements for referral, assessment and management. Purchasers should monitor local arrangements and ensure adequate controls are in place.

- Where the service is defined as exceeding the requirements of general medical services, following consultation and agreement with the profession, the question of additional payment for the delivery of a specialist service needs to be considered.

The concept of harm minimization

As drug-taking becomes more frequent, so the likelihood increases that medical, social, psychological or legal problems will develop. The harm caused by these problems affects not only individual drug misusers, but also their family and friends and the population that lives nearby, whether or not they are acquainted with the drug taker concerned. It is now widely recognized that harm associated with these problems can be minimized by appropriate professional input and that this is a much more constructive approach than treatments that aim at chemical abstinence alone. The way forward needs to be on a broad front, with appropriate co-ordinated professional input into the social, psychological, criminal and medical aspects of drug taking.

This is best done as a partnership approach, not only for the treatment of individual drug misusers by shared-care arrangements, but also on a locality basis by locality action groups, and more widely still at District chief officer level, through the work of drug action teams. Some of the medical harm to individual drug misusers can be minimized by GPs through the provision of general medical services and further harm minimization can be achieved either by referral to, or working together with, specialist drug services.

Nevertheless, many GPs have concerns over their roles when a drug misuser attends the surgery asking for help. What is the most

appropriate help for them to provide and where do their responsibilities end under general medical services? These concerns are
addressed throughout this book and are at first best viewed in the
context of developments that have taken place in UK national policy.

Historical developments

In 1912, Britain signed the Hague Convention and in doing so gave
an international commitment to control the supply of certain narcotic
and other drugs. The first defined legislation on drugs of dependence
in the UK, the Dangerous Drugs Act, followed in 1920. This Act allowed doctors to use narcotic drugs for bona fide medical treatment,
but unfortunately did not state whether this included the treatment
of drug dependence. A Departmental Committee on Morphine and
Heroin Addicts was set up to sort out this issue and was chaired by
Sir Humphrey Rolleston, the then President of the Royal College of
Physicians. The Departmental Committee's deliberations were published in 1926 and became known as the Rolleston report.[6] This was
the first defined policy on the treatment of drug dependence in the
UK. It was a flexible policy and was envied by physicians in many
other countries, such as the USA, where a doctor's clinical freedom
to treat opiate addicts in the way he or she felt was most appropriate
was curtailed by restrictive legislation. The Rolleston report outlined
the following two indications for the use of morphine or heroin in the
treatment of drug dependence:

* if the person was being gradually withdrawn

* if, after attempts at cure had failed, the patient could lead a
  normal and useful life when provided with a regular supply, but
  ceased to do so when the supply was withdrawn.

Thus the principle of maintenance treatment was born and this
became known as 'the British system'. The number of opiate addicts
in the UK at that time was relatively small. Before the 1950s, there were
so few heroin addicts in Britain that nearly all of them were known
personally to the Home Office Drugs Branch Inspectorate, which
periodically checked pharmacy records.[7] There were several exaggerated press reports about the danger to the British public of Chinese
opium dens in London's docklands, but in reality almost all opiate

dependent people in the UK were the victims of unnecessarily prolonged prescribing of morphine by their doctors. Often these patients
had been treated with morphine for a physically painful condition,
and had found serendipitous relief for an emotionally painful condition, e.g. an anxiety state. Then when the pain disappeared they
resisted the cessation of their opiate prescription. From 1926 until the
late 1950s, the number of people who were being helped to lead
normal and useful lives through the 'British system' (usually on an
injectable morphine prescription) was stable, varying between 400
and 600. These people were mainly middle class and middle aged,
or elderly.

The Brain Committee reports

Around 1960, reports began to emerge of a new group of opiate drug
takers. These were young people, mainly in their late teens and twenties, who were misusing and advocating the use of prescribed drugs for
'kicks'. An Interdepartmental Committee on Drug Addiction chaired
by Sir Russell Brain was set up to look into this matter, and reported
in 1961 that the drug situation in Britain gave little cause for concern.[8] However, media coverage continued and the committee was
asked to reconvene. In 1965, the second Brain Committee reported
very differently that a new, young, unstable, non-therapeutic group of
drug takers had emerged, and that although some illicitly produced
drugs were sold on the street, most of the problem was caused through
overprescribing of therapeutic drugs by unscrupulous, uninformed,
or vulnerable doctors open to blackmail.[9] The second Brain Committee recommended that where possible prescribing should be taken
out of the hands of GPs and instead carried out by specialist psychiatrists, who would work from special centres to be known as drug
dependence units (DDUs).

The DDUs were set up between 1968–70 in densely populated
inner-city areas, mainly in London. They were few in number and
almost exclusively confined to England. Only one specialist centre
for drug users was established in Wales, and none at all in Scotland
and Northern Ireland. Since not all areas of the country could be cov-
ered by the new breed of specialist psychiatrists, general psychiatrists
and GPs, although discouraged, were not completely prevented from
treating drug misusers. However, heavy penalties were put in place
for any doctor who prescribed inappropriately or excessively. As a

consequence the treatment of drug addiction by doctors who were not specialist psychiatrists virtually stopped, and many people were optimistic that this 'new' problem would go away.

It did not go away, indeed methadone prescribed by the DDUs became a new street drug, and throughout the 1970s the number of known drug addicts continued to rise slowly. Then in the late 1970s there was a sudden very rapid increase in the numbers of known opiate users. There were several reasons for this:

• cheap and plentiful supplies of illicitly produced heroin from abundant harvests in Pakistan and the Far East

• the appeal of high-gain, low-risk operations enticed criminal gangs (who had previously avoided this area of activity) to start drug trafficking

• the widespread introduction of the then new habit of smoking heroin ('chasing the dragon') as opposed to injecting or sniffing it.

After almost two decades, in spite of many efforts to contain it, a relentless increase in illicit drug use has continued, particularly among young people. Every year the situation has worsened, in the UK and throughout the world. During this time many changes have taken place in the UK. The rapid increase in numbers of opiate users seeking help caused the specialist services to become overwhelmed. The British system of maintenance prescribing was questioned, and by the early 1980s all the specialist clinics, without exception, moved over to rigid detoxification regimens of a maximum duration of three to six months.

The changing role of the GP

Changes that affected GPs began in 1982 when once again they were invited to play a role in the field. In its report *Treatment and Rehabilitation*,[10] the Advisory Council on the Misuse of Drugs (ACMD) stated: 'Given the widening geographical distribution of problem drug taking and the increased variety of drugs misused, we are aware that it would be unreasonable to expect future hospital services to be developed to the point where they could provide comprehensive cover in all districts, particularly where access to specialist services is poor. We see therefore a possible role for some doctors outside the specialist services to play a part in the treatment of problem drug takers, but with strict safeguards'. This was followed in 1984 by the publication of *Guidelines of Good Clinical Practice in the Treatment of Drug Misuse* by the Department of Health (DoH). The document included guidelines for GPs and had the backing of both the British Medical Association (BMA) and the General Medical Services Committee (GMSC). It stated: 'General practitioners are increasingly likely to see patients presenting with drug related problems in view of the increasing incidence of opioid addiction. We wish to encourage as many general practitioners as possible to treat these patients and to help them in every possible way ...'. Since that time successive official policy documents have stressed the importance of involving GPs in the treatment process.

General practitioners have, however, not been quick to come forward, and this has not been from a lack of opiate users asking them for help. In a national survey of GPs and the treatment of opiate misuse published in 1985,[11] Glanz estimated that between 30 000 and 40 000 new cases of opiate misuse presented to GPs each year, and that a typical GP in England and Wales with a list of 2000 patients will have about two new cases of opiate misuse in a year. Several GPs in the survey stated they would probably play a more active part in the treatment of opiate misusers if more back-up resources were available.

The impact of HIV

Events then took an unforeseen change. It became clear that Britain was facing an epidemic of human immunodeficiency virus (HIV) infection with enormous social and financial implications, and that the all-important predicted third wave of heterosexual spread of the disease would enter the general heterosexual population, mainly through index cases who were drug users. Something had to be done quickly and a working party of the ACMD was set up in 1987 to report on the issues and to make recommendations. The first of three reports on acquired immune deficiency syndrome (AIDS) and drug misuse was published in 1988.[12] It was highly influential and led to a major change in the way that drug services worked with clients. The report stated as a fundamental principle that it was more important to both the individual and the public health to limit the spread of HIV within the drug-using population than to overcome the drug problem itself. Harm reduction was to take precedence over abstinence, and although abstinence was not to be lost sight of, there was a hierarchy of other goals that were more important to achieve. An example of this hierarchy for an individual drug misuser might be:

1   the cessation of sharing injecting equipment
2   the cessation of injecting
3   reduction of drug use
4   abstinence.

It was now important to be proactive rather than reactive so that services could reach as many drug users as possible, including those who did not wish to stop using drugs, to help them reduce the risk of contracting and spreading HIV disease both through shared injecting practices and sexually. It was recommended that outreach services and facilities for the promotion of needle exchange be introduced. General practitioners were seen as a key resource because of their widespread accessibility and because they would be one of the first ports of call when drug problems began to develop. They were thus in a good position to reduce the spread of HIV at an early stage, both by giving harm-reduction advice, and by prescribing oral opiate substitute drugs, such as methadone mixture to opiate injectors.

One of the recommendations was to give more back-up resources to GPs by the provision of community drugs teams (CDTs) in every health district. The teams would work with GPs on a shared-care basis. The CDTs would perform a counselling and non-prescribing function and the GP would look after the medical side of the treatment package. The teams would be a source of expert advice for GPs, if required, and would work closely with GPs on individual cases. This package of measures is now recognized as having been highly successful in helping to limit the epidemic of HIV in drug users and reducing its spread into the general heterosexual population.[13] The prevalence rate of HIV-1 in current injectors living in London was found to have stabilized at 7% in multi-site studies from 1990–93.[14] More recently data from the third unlinked anonymous survey of HIV infection in England and Wales have shown a decline. At 1.5%, infection rates among injecting drug users in London in 1995 were half those in 1994.[15] The prevalence rate among current injectors in England outside of London has remained low at less than 1%.[15] In Scotland the prevalence rate was 1% in Glasgow in 1992,[16] and the previously high levels in Edinburgh had dropped in 1994 to about 20%.[17] There is, however, no room for complacency particularly as a much larger epidemic of hepatitis C has surfaced. Six out of every ten users with a history of injecting who attend UK drug services are hepatitis C-positive.[18] These figures cover not just opiate users who inject, but also injectors of a wide variety of other drugs including amphetamine, cocaine and benzodiazepines.

Drug use statistics

- About one in six (18%) of the UK population has taken a drug sometime in their life. This is around nine million people[19]

- In any year, at least 6% of the UK population will take an illegal drug – some three million people[19]

- A survey of 5000 people aged 16 and over in four UK cities showed that 36% of 16–19 year olds and 41% of 20–24 year olds had taken illicit drugs[20]

- A three-year study in the North-West of England reported that by the last year of the study when most of the people surveyed were aged 16, the majority (51%) said they had taken illicit drugs[21]

- About 15% of adults surveyed,[20] and nearly a quarter of 16–29 year olds[22] admit to having tried cannabis

- There appears to have been a rapid increase in the use of cannabis by young people. Exeter University in an annual survey[23] of 50 000 schoolchildren reported that of 14–15 year olds:

  – 2% said they had tried cannabis in 1988

  – 16% said they had tried it in 1993

  – 23% said they had tried it in 1994

- The prevalence of opioid injecting among adults is now reported to be 1–2% in some inner cities in the UK[24]

Patterns of drug use

Drug use varies throughout the UK. Opiates are the most commonly notified drug of misuse. In general, benzodiazepine misuse increases northwards from England to Scotland, particularly the misuse of temazepam, so that for GPs in Scotland problems from temazepam misuse are frequently seen. Drug misuse in Northern Ireland has remained consistently low, in contrast to the rest of the UK and Southern Ireland. Crack cocaine is becoming an increasing problem, particularly in urban areas. Amphetamine, which had previously been found mainly in rural areas, is now used everywhere. The 1990s have seen the emergence of the dance-drug culture with Ecstasy, amphetamine and amyl nitrite (a drug previously used almost exclusively by homosexuals) widely used by both sexes at raves, nightclubs and discos. Cannabis is in extremely common use throughout Britain. Anabolic steroid use is also causing concern.

Drugs that are commonly misused

Cannabis

Opioids, e.g. heroin, morphine, dihydrocodeine, buprenorphine

CNS depressant drugs, e.g. benzodiazepines, barbiturates, alcohol

CNS stimulant drugs, e.g. amphetamine, cocaine and the hallucinogenic amphetamines (such as Ecstasy)

Psychedelic drugs, e.g. LSD, magic mushrooms

Volatile substances, e.g. glue, lighter fuel, petrol, aerosols

Other drugs, e.g. cyclizine, amyl nitrite, anabolic steroids

As a result of medical or other problems related to drug misuse, GPs may come in contact with misusers of a wide variety of drugs, often at a relatively early stage in their drug-taking career. It is those GPs, who have developed skills to deal with drug users, who are in a good position to facilitate change. Of paramount importance is a constructive doctor–patient relationship. General practitioners do not need to know every small detail of every drug of misuse. This book will demystify and give insights on how to handle misusers of different groups of drugs, but drug problems are essentially people problems, and the knowledge and skills that GPs have developed to help their other patients with problems will be of most help. Substitute prescribing, if it is needed, is an easily learnt technique, and is usually best done on a shared-care basis with the local drug service, which will act as a source of expert advice and support. Treating drug misusers can be a heavy burden on time, but with realistic expectations, reducing harm to both the individual and the local community through small, progressive goals makes it well worthwhile. Working in a general practice setting to help a young person minimize the harm from drug dependence, earning the deep-felt gratitude of the person concerned, their family and close friends can be a very rewarding experience.

Increasing GP involvement

In spite of the setting up of CDTs on a national basis, the involvement of GPs in the treatment of drug dependence has been patchy and slow. There are a few areas of the country, such as Edinburgh, where GP involvement has been good, but many others where it is virtually non-existent. This is not surprising given the lack of undergraduate and postgraduate medical education in this field, coupled with the knowledge that a doctor can be hauled before a tribunal and even struck off for wrongful prescribing. The message that GPs should avoid this area of work, hammered home so effectively after the second Brain Committee report, has lingered on in the minds of many doctors. Lack of education on the subject has led to biased attitudes. Yet some GPs are providing an exemplary service and their professional help has been greatly appreciated by drug users and their families. General practitioners who work in this way are slowly increasing in number, but not at a rate that is fast enough to contain the problem.

One way forward was initiated in Glasgow in 1993.[25] This was to pay GPs for providing a specialist service for the treatment of opiate drug dependence. The type of treatment for which pay would be given was defined, and GPs were expected to undergo preliminary training to enable them to enrol for the scheme. In Glasgow payment was made for GPs running clinics for opiate drug users because originally the funding was provided under the aegis of running them as health promotion clinics. Later in Edinburgh and several other places, specific payments were made by health boards (or in England, NHS health authorities) for the treatment of individual drug users. There are many different models.

Clearly such payments can only be made for work over and above what is expected through ordinary general medical services (GMS). At a Royal College of GPs conference on managing drug users in general practice in 1996, the following consensus statement was agreed:[26]

• all GPs should offer GMS to drug users

• all GPs should be willing to assess drug misuse problems and refer patients as appropriate

• where GPs take on an extended role in the care of drug users this should be resourced in recognition of the extra workload involved

• there is an urgent need for training about drug misuse to be included in 'core medical training' at an undergraduate level. There is also a need for continuing medical education in this area for all GP registrars, GPs and hospital doctors.

The recognition that some GPs who had gained special expertise in working with drug users should be paid an extra sum of money paved the way to the development of a suggested new contract where GPs could be paid additional amounts for doing other areas of work that also required special training over and above core general medical services.[27] The implementation of this new contract could encourage many more GPs from all over the country to receive appropriate training in the treatment of problem drug use. In addition, locally agreed protocols and guidelines should lead to substantially more GPs becoming involved in high-quality professional treatment of drug misusers. A potential workforce of 32 000 GPs would make a significant impact on the problem.

2

Assessment of the drug user

Chris Ford and Brian Whitehead

General practitioners and primary health care teams are increasingly likely to be consulted by drug users and are a first point of contact for many.[1] General practice is in a unique position to provide services to whole families and GPs are ideally located to respond to a wide variety of their needs. General practitioners see a broader and more varied range of drug users than many of the specialist treatment services that have traditionally focused on long-term opiate users.

Assessment is the mutual gathering of information to ascertain patients' needs and to assist in defining the most appropriate course of action. Decisions about the treatment of individual patients should be based as far as possible on a thorough assessment of what will work for that person and on reliable information on what works generally.

Benefits of a comprehensive assessment

- Allows a profile of the client, and the client's drug problem to be developed

- Helps drug users to think about why they use drugs and what they may need to change

- Helps identify the client's health and social needs

- Helps identify the most appropriate treatment

- Helps identify treatment goals, such as stability of lifestyle and a move away from crime

- Helps decide whether this patient can/should be treated by the GP in general practice. This will be informed by:

    - the experience of the GP

    - relationships with local services

    - the ability to refer to additional services

Levels of GP involvement

General practitioners need to consider what level of involvement with drug users is appropriate for them and their practice. They also need to consider the extent of their competence and ability before they become involved in certain aspects of the treatment of drug users, such as substitute prescribing.

Possible levels of GP involvement[2]

1   No provision of services to known illicit drug users

2   Provision of GMS only

3   Provision of drug-related interventions under direct super-vision

4   Provision of drug-related interventions with specialist support as required

5   The specialist GP

Taking on long-term dependent heroin users is a totally different pro-position to providing advice to a recreational weekend Ecstasy user. There are likely to be a number of problems of a physical, psy-chological and social nature in those drug users who have been using illicit drugs for longer periods. Chaotic long-term polydrug users with mental health issues are amongst the most complicated of patients to manage and may be completely out of the range of many GPs, except for their general health care.

Accept your limits

- Are you able to commit to an increased workload and consultation time?

- Are you prepared to work long term with drug users, perhaps over many years, to effect change?

Define your philosophy

- Are you clear and comfortable with the philosophy of treatment/care that influences your interventions?

- Are you clear about your aims? (Abstinence or maintenance.)

Match philosophy to patients

- Is your philosophy compatible with the needs of your patients?

Factors to consider before deciding to treat a drug user
in general practice

1 *Type of drug use*: Is drug use experimental or recreational? Non-problematic drug use may not require prescribing.

2 *Duration of drug use*: Is duration of drug use short or medium term? Shorter-term drug use is more manageable. However, given experience and support, long-term drug users can be managed in general practice.[3]

3 *Drug type(s)*: Using only one drug? Usually opiate, cocaine or amphetamine.

   Polydrug use? Usually heroin or methadone with or without benzodiazepines.

4 *Quantity of drug*: Less than 1 g heroin or 60 mg diazepam daily?

5 *Social*: Some social support available? Partner, family or friends? Non-using partner or friends?

6 *Housing*: Suitable and secure?

7 *Criminal*: In a cycle of crime to fund habit?

8   *Health status compromised by drug use?* Consider medical conditions, e.g. HIV infection/hepatitis C.

9   *Dual diagnosis*: If patient is frankly mentally ill, may not be suitable for GP care alone.

10   *Address*: Needs to live in practice area.

Patients who may need referral to statutory agencies

- Need high degree of intervention and/or counselling
- Need help with other problems: housing, benefits
- Have concurrent mental illness
- Other addictions, e.g. alcohol
- Using a combination of different drugs

Assessment by the GP in surgery

An assessment of a drug user seeking help will assist in the formulation of an appropriate treatment plan. A full assessment can take place over several consultations to fit in with normal surgeries.

At assessment the GP needs to be able to:

1   Establish that the patient is using drugs and the type of drug use – experimental, recreational or dependent. At the same time, offer brief interventions that provide specific advice on risk reduction and harm minimization.

2   Identify what drugs, by what administration route and reasons for use. (Assess the amounts being taken and degree of dependence.)

3   Identify what problems and concerns the patient has.

4   Assess the patient's motivation in relation to these problems and concerns.

5   Determine if the patient's drug use is causing concurrent physical/psychological/social problems.

There is rarely a need to decide on treatment at the first visit. Patients do not die from withdrawals and taking time to assess and formulate a treatment plan is better than being forced into prescribing immediately.

Waiting allows time for:

- the name and address of the patient to be verified

- proof of local residency to be provided

- urine screen results to arrive (although this is sometimes impractical in areas where there is a delay with processing)

- the drug user to decide that treatment is wanted

- the GP to decide if this user can be managed in general practice.

Levels of intervention with drug users

Type of use

Experimental/recreational

Dependent:
a) long-term chaotic
b) polydrug use
c) dual diagnosis
d) pregnant drug user

Level of intervention

Minimal:
brief intervention

High:
long-term care

Provision of services

GMS
Harm minimization/health
    promotion
Advice/information
Assessment/referral

Prescribing
Stabilisation
Maintenance
    Reduction
    Detoxification
Relapse prevention
Referral to/from specialist
    agency
In-patient detoxification
Residential rehabilitation

The assessment process

1 Why has the patient presented now?

- Why has the patient come to you?
- Why now? Is there a legal problem? Have they been sent by friends, family, probation, or are they coming for themselves?
- What do they want? (It will not always be drugs.)
- What do they see as the problem?
- What do you see as the problem?
- Are you willing to help with their drug problem?
- Are you willing to help with any other health and social problems?

2 How has the patient presented?

- Outside surgery hours.
- With an arranged appointment.
- With a friend who is registered.
- As an emergency.
- As a temporary resident.
- In obvious withdrawals.

3 How does the patient seem?

- Drowsy, elated, restless.
- Having difficulty in concentrating.
- Unkempt appearance.
- Inconsistent in their story.

4 Are there indications of drug use?

- Trackmarks – new/old.

- Pupils dilated or constricted.

- Tremor, weight loss.

5 Assessment of drug use

- What drugs have been taken in the past month? Current drugs being used? What is their primary drug? What is their current level of use?

- How much and how often?

- Route of use? (Oral, smoking, skin-popping, intravenous?)

- Are any drugs being prescribed or not?

- Withdrawal symptoms?

- Evidence of recent drug use, e.g. abscesses, injection sites, intoxication?

6 Drug history

- At what age did the user start taking drugs (including alcohol and cannabis)?

- When did drug taking become a problem?

- What was the progression from one type of drug to another?

- What combination of drugs have been used?

- What are the reasons for one drug over another?

- Has the drug user ever been abstinent from the drug of choice? When and for how long?

- If yes, how was this possible?

- What level of control do they have over their use?

7 Previous treatments

- Has the drug user had previous treatments?

- Have treatments been in-patient, rehabilitation, specialist, GP?

- When and for how long?

- Did they achieve abstinence and for how long?

- Why did they relapse?

- What worked/did not work for them?

- Why are they returning for treatment now?

8 Assessing risk taking behaviour

- Do they ever inject? Are they injecting safely?

- Have they shared/lent needles or syringes? (Regularly, occasionally, frequently?)

- Have they shared any drug-using paraphernalia, such as filters or spoons?

- Where do they obtain their equipment? (Needle exchange, pharmacy?)

- What are their current cleaning techniques?

- Are they currently in a sexual relationship? (Regular, casual, both?)

- What is the sex of their partner/s?

- Do they practise safe or unsafe sex?

- Do they use condoms and, if so, from where do they obtain them?

- Are they aware of HIV infection, hepatitis B and C and how these viruses are transmitted?

9 Assessment of physical and psychological health

- Any medical problems? (Acute, chronic.)

- Any drug-related medical problems? (Abscesses, thrombosis, septicaemia, fits, hepatitis B, hepatitis C, HIV.)

- Is the drug user on any medication?

- Is the drug user depressed?

- Any other psychiatric disorder present?

10 Assessment of social situation

- *Personal relationships*: partner, family, friends, children
  - using/non-using partner; using/non-using friends
  - contact with family
  - do they have children; how many, ages, and where and with whom do they live?
- *Accommodation*: stable/homeless
  - type: private rented, council, housing association, own, squat
  - problems with housing: crowded, damp, unsuitable.
- *Employment history*: What/how long/casual or not?
  - short/long term; qualifications; hopes for employment.
- *Legal situation*: History of offences. Is there a current court case pending?
  - periods in prison. Does the drug user have a probation officer?
- *Financial situation*: Income from benefits/work; debts
  - how is drug habit financed? (Remember confidentiality and explain.)

Goal setting

- Important to identify goals so that treatment has direction and focus
- Goals need to be identified collaboratively with the patient so that both parties are clear about what is to be achieved
- Goals should be specific, attainable and measurable
- Goals should start with the areas of risk: reducing illicit drug use, reducing levels of injecting and sharing
- Help patient to think about how these changes may be brought about
- Assessment should be sequential and on-going: build upon previous work
- Set a review date within a week or so

Urine screening

A urine drug screen is an essential safeguard and helpful tool that should always be obtained at the outset of treatment, and randomly through the course of treatment. 50 ml of urine is required.

Why do urine screens?

- To confirm that patient is using drugs and which ones.
- To help decide on the treatment plan.
- For your medico-legal protection.
- For the patient's protection.
- To help reduce street diversion.
- To help identify the hoarder.
- To encourage honesty – repeat if very different from patient's story. (Mistakes at the laboratory are possible.)

When asked, a group of users in Glasgow said they valued having their urine tested because it showed someone cared enough to bother to check their story.

What does a urine test show?

1   The range of drugs being used.

2   It is a qualitative test, *not* a quantitative measure.

3   If the user is dependent – opiates persist in urine up to 24 hours, methadone up to 48 hours. If the urine test result is negative and there is no evidence of withdrawing, the user is not dependent.

When to do a urine screen

1   When a drug user presents (even if you are not going to pre-scribe), as a useful baseline or for future comparisons.

2   To confirm use before starting a substitute prescription.

3   Before restarting a script after a break in treatment, or a relapse.

4   At random throughout treatment to check on drug use against stated use.

Approximate drug detection times in urine

Heroin/morphine	1–3 days (possibly only one day)
Methadone	1–2 days (very dose dependent)
Dihydrocodeine	4–5 days (in high concentration)
Codeine	2–3 days
Pholcodeine	10–15 days
Amphetamines	1–2 days (can be detected up to 4 days)
Cocaine	12 hours–3 days
Benzodiazepines	1 day–3 weeks (acute or chronic use)
Barbiturates	days–weeks (depending on type)
Cannabis – casual use	2–7 days
– heavy use	up to 30 days
Ecstasy	2–4 days
Buprenorphine	2–3 days
Alcohol	12–24 hours

Factors affecting drug detection times

1   The drug.

2   The quantity of drug taken.

3   Single dose or chronic use.

4   Other drugs taken.

5   Taken with alcohol (enzyme inducer, increases metabolic rate which removes the prime drug faster).

6   The concentration of urine (the reason why a creatinine is measured concurrently).

Initial screens are done by immunoassay, which lacks the specificity of the older chromatographic techniques. As a result, a positive opiate immunoassay may not find a low level of morphine when present with other metabolites. The methadone assay is designed to detect just the parent drug and not the metabolite. Hence the detection time is short and can be used to check consumption of a daily dose. Some specialist services have their own screening facilities. It may be possible to make an arrangement to use them. Highly sensitive dipsticks for commonly misused substances, e.g. heroin, methadone, are increasingly available.

Notification

Until the end of April 1997, doctors were legally required to notify the Home Office if they knew or suspected a patient was using one of 14 notifiable drugs (13 were opiate drugs and the other cocaine). This requirement has now been abolished. As a result, the Addicts Index, where details of notifications were recorded, has also ceased to exist. Doctors can no longer use this Index to ascertain if a patient they are seeing has been recently prescribed for by another doctor.

Notification to the local Regional Drug Misuse Database should continue to be made. A wide range of drug use should be notified, including the use of many non-opiate drugs of addiction. Notification is voluntary and can be made by workers from drug agencies as well as doctors. The information is confidential as neither the name nor address of the drug user is included. Notification is only of users 'newly presenting' to an agency within a six-month period, and therefore provides information about trends in drug use rather than monitoring individuals.

3

General health care of drug users

Katie Kemp

Introduction

A trebling in the number of substance misusers notified to the Home Office over the last decade[1] means that most GPs can expect to see an increased demand for help from those using illicit drugs. Whether or not a GP feels able to treat the drug dependency itself, few would disagree that GPs have an important role in providing general medical care to drug users, and over the last ten years the DoH has increasingly encouraged GPs to do so.[2] There is evidence that substance misusers would prefer to receive treatment for their drug dependency from their GPs[3] and that drug users registered with a GP consult their doctor more frequently than non drug-using patients.[4,5] This places GPs in a key position to detect and treat ill health in substance misusers and provides opportunities to screen for infectious and transmissible disease, vaccinate against preventable diseases, such as hepatitis A and B, and to educate about the risks associated with illicit drug use.

Morbidity and mortality are greatly increased in people who misuse drugs, especially those injecting drugs and practising unsafe sex.[6] Accepting substance misusers onto their lists may significantly increase demands upon GPs' time and medical skills. The illnesses to which many drug users succumb include all forms of viral hepatitis, bacterial endocarditis, HIV, tuberculosis, septicaemia, pneumonia, deep venous thrombosis, pulmonary emboli and abscesses, to name but a few. The difficulty for the GP is that many of the serious infections that may commonly occur in intravenous drug users are now generally uncommon in the rest of the population. This may hinder our ability to recognize illnesses that we rarely see and have little experience in treating. Despite the difficulties and increased workload involved, GPs report positively on their experience of providing treatment to drug users.[7,8]

Assessing the physical health of the drug user

Table 3.1: Health assessment

Elicit from the history	Note on examination	Investigate
• What drug(s) are used? • How much drug is used? • Frequency of use? • Route of administration? – sharing injecting equipment? • Duration of use? • Previous treatment? • Current health problems? • Past medical history? – abscesses/cellulitis – hepatitis – bacterial endocarditis – septicaemia – deep venous thrombosis – tuberculosis – HIV – venous ulcers • Social circumstances? – accommodation – employment/income – family/social support – legal difficulties • Vaccinated for hepatitis B? • Safe sex/contraception?	• General – undue drowsiness – high arousal – signs of withdrawal – self-neglect • Height/weight • Skin – abscesses – injecting sites – venous ulcers – anaemia – parasites – self-mutilation • Chest – chest infections – cardiac murmurs – wheeze • Abdomen – hepatomegaly – splenomegaly – constipation – pregnancy – groin sinuses	• Urine – drugs being abused? • Full blood count – anaemia? – raised MCV? • Liver function – gamma GT? – other enzymes? • Hepatitis B – antibodies? – carrier status? – non-immune? • Consider counselling and screening for: – HIV and hepatitis C • Pregnancy test needed if amenorrhoea is present • Cervical cytology • STD screen

Source: Kemp K and Orr M (1996) Managing Drug Misusers – a guide. *The Practitioner*. **240**: 326–34.

It is helpful to make a full assessment of the substance misuser's general health as early as possible after acceptance onto the list. Although time constraints in a busy surgery may tempt the GP to avoid investing a large amount of time in an often unplanned consultation, the benefits of a thorough history, examination and pertinent investigations are manifold.

- Many intravenous drug users may have chequered medical and social histories, with frequent previous changes of GP and address. Medical records 'following' such patients can at best be incomplete and at worst unobtainable.

- A history of drug-taking activity and the patient's past and current medical problems can help to determine the most appropriate treatment options, as well as enabling the detection of significant ill health.

- A baseline of the patient's current health can be established, from which future deviations may alert the GP to the development of new disease processes.

- A careful medical assessment can provide the opportunity to offer appropriate vaccines and to discuss HIV and hepatitis screening.

- Finally, a thorough assessment of the substance misuser's health and lifestyle demonstrates interest in the patient and may help to dispel the fear of rejection that many drug users anticipate from health professionals.[9]

A comprehensive assessment can be performed over several consultations if necessary, particularly if the patient is returning to the surgery regularly for substitute prescribing.

Clinical examination

Substance misusers may not immediately declare their illicit drug use to the GP. Some fear judgemental attitudes, breach of confidentiality or are ashamed of their habit. Consequently, the diagnosis of drug use may not be considered until physical examination is undertaken. Intoxication with drugs or alcohol, poor levels of general education, lack of awareness of the possible cause of their ill health and reticence born of mistrust can conspire to make some drug abusers poor historians whose symptomatology is at best vague and not uncommonly masked by the substances they are using. Clinical examination of any substance misuser (suspected or declared) is therefore of paramount importance and is often more illuminating than the

history. In addition to the observations that a doctor routinely notes
during examination of any patient, it may be helpful to consider the
following when examining a known or suspected drug user.

1 General state

- Look for evidence of withdrawal from opiates, such as increased
  lacrimation, rhinorrhoea, sweating, pilo-erection, dilated pupils
  and raised blood pressure.

- Conversely, undue drowsiness and pin-point pupils may indicate
  very recent opiate use.

- Agitation or high arousal may indicate stimulant use or withdrawal from opiates.

- Self-neglect and homelessness are common in those heavily
  addicted to drugs, and patients may often appear unkempt.

- Cocaine and amphetamines cause anorexia and their use may
  result in significant weight loss.

- Generalized lymphadenopathy may be present in HIV-positive
  patients.

- Pyrexia above 38°C may indicate the presence of significant
  underlying infection, and septicaemia should be considered in
  those injecting drug users in whom no other discernible cause for
  fever is found.

2 Examination of the skin

- This may reveal the presence of stigmata, such as scars from old
  abscesses and 'trackmarks'. The latter appear as discolorations of
  the skin overlying commonly used injection sites and are patho-
  gnomonic of intravenous drug use.

- Localized abscesses, cellulitis and superficial thrombophlebitis
  are all commonly observed on inspection of the skin in injecting
  drug users and may provide important clues as to the source of
  sepsis in those patients presenting with generalized septicaemia,
  acute endocarditis or bone and joint infections.

- Venous ulceration and/or oedema of the lower limbs is often seen
  and may be caused by chronic venous insufficiency resulting
  from recurrent deep venous thromboses.

- Inspection of injecting sites can be helpful and may reveal the presence of sinuses (commonly found over the femoral veins in those injecting into the groin) which can provide potential sources of infection.

- Palmar erythema and spider telangiectasia may be present in those patients with liver disease, and jaundice may be noted in patients with acute hepatitis A or B or in those with liver failure secondary to chronic active hepatitis.

- Rashes are most commonly attributable to parasites such as scabies, but the presence of a diffuse maculo-papular rash in an unwell intravenous drug user should alert the GP to the possibility of a seroconversion illness associated with exposure to HIV.

- Transient skin rashes may also occur in the prodromal phase of hepatitis B.

- Small areas of infarcted skin may result from crack/cocaine use[10] and bacterial endocarditis can produce splinter haemorrhages under the fingernails and petechial haemorrhages in the skin and mucous membranes.

- Scarring from self-mutilation is frequently seen, reflecting the high incidence of psychiatric co-morbidity amongst substance misusers.

3 Assessment of the chest and cardiovascular system

Examination of the chest and cardiovascular system in the sick intravenous drug user may provide a variety of useful diagnostic signs associated with any of the following conditions.

- Most intravenous drug users smoke cigarettes and the incidence of bronchitis, obstructive airways disease and tumours of the lung is high.

- Intravenous drug users also have an increased incidence of bacterial pneumonia and tuberculosis.

- HIV-positive drug users are not only particularly susceptible to both of the latter but also to opportunist chest infections, such as pneumocystis pneumoniae.

- Inhalation of cocaine has been associated with atelectasis, alveolar haemorrhage and pulmonary oedema, and may provoke constriction of the coronary arteries producing anginal symptoms.

- Both cocaine and amphetamine abuse can cause tachycardia and arrhythmias.

- Injecting drug users may develop pheumothoraces, pulmonary emboli, bacterial endocarditis and aspiration pneumonias.

A cardiac murmur in an unwell intravenous drug user should be regarded as suspicious and investigated accordingly. The GP's threshold for requesting a chest X-ray should be suitably low if any significant chest infection is suspected.

4 Abdominal examination

- Palpation of the abdomen often demonstrates the presence of constipation in heroin or methadone users since opiates reduce gut motility.

- Hepatic enlargement may indicate an acute hepatitis or heavy alcohol intake.

- An enlarged spleen can occur during seroconversion following exposure to HIV, is commonly found in bacterial endocarditis, and may also be present in early stages of hepatitis.

- Epigastric tenderness may indicate acute gastritis or peptic ulceration, both of which occur more commonly in substance misusers who ingest large quantities of alcohol, smoke heavily and have poor eating habits.

- Pancreatitis, both acute and chronic, can produce few symptoms other than vague abdominal pain and nausea but is not uncommon amongst drug users who also consume alcohol.

- Lower abdominal tenderness in female drug users may indicate pelvic inflammatory disease. Occasionally abdominal palpation reveals a gravid uterus in an amenorrhoeic drug user who has not suspected that she is pregnant.

5 The musculo-skeletal system

- Injecting drug users frequently complain of muscular aches and pains, arthralgia and bone pain.

- Sometimes these symptoms are manifestations of the withdrawal syndrome but it should be remembered that the prodromal phases of hepatitis A and B can produce similar symptomatology, as can bacterial endocarditis.

- Septic arthritis and infective osteomyelitis occur more commonly in those who inject drugs.

- Rhabdomyolysis has been reported secondary to both heroin and cocaine use, but is relatively rare.

6 The central nervous system

- Many substance misusers report 'fits' and the incidence of epileptiform seizures is increased in patients withdrawing from both benzodiazepines and alcohol.

- Convulsions may also occur in association with cocaine toxicity. True idiopathic or inherent epilepsy should nevertheless be excluded.

- Cerebral abscesses resulting from septic emboli and candida ophthalmitis (the latter often presenting as a painful red eye) also occur more frequently in those injecting drugs.

- Peripheral neuropathy may be noted in chronic alcohol abusers and may also result from the inhalation of volatile substances, such as butane.

- HIV-positive substance misusers may also present with cerebral toxoplasmosis, cryptococcal meningitis, cerebral lymphoma or any other of the well-documented neurological manifestations associated with HIV infection.

Health of female drug users

Sexual health

Many women support their drug habit by prostitution and therefore contract chlamydia, gonorrhoea and other sexually transmitted diseases more readily than the non-drug using population. Even those women not 'street-working' are at an increased risk of contracting venereal diseases because safer sexual practices are not widespread amongst drug users. Pelvic examination and high vaginal and endocervical swabs should be performed in female drug users complaining of vaginal discharge, lower abdominal pain or urinary tract symptoms. Referral to a genito-urinary medicine clinic can be offered (and provides invaluable help with contract tracing should this be necessary) although not all patients will accept this, and even those who do will not always attend once appointments have been made.

Both prostitution and the increased prevalence of HIV amongst intravenous drug users significantly increase the risk of cervical intra-epithelial neoplasia (CIN) in women who use drugs.[11] Human papilloma virus and herpes virus are also more commonly found in drug users. Cervical cytological screening therefore reveals a much higher incidence of abnormalities amongst substance misusers and it is worthwhile performing a smear on all female drug users as part of an overall health assessment. Although some patients will express anxiety about pelvic examination (there is extensive research establishing a high incidence of childhood sexual abuse amongst drug users) it should be remembered that the intravenous drug user's lifestyle and irregular contact with medical services means that they are much more likely to slip through the conventional screening net.

Contraception

Contraception can also be discussed during sexual health screening. A large number of female patients using opiates will complain of amenorrhoea and many of these will assume that they are therefore infertile and do not require contraception. The increased prevalence of hepatitis B and C (and associated liver damage), alcohol abuse, tuberculosis, HIV, amenorrhoea and history of deep venous thrombosis, combined with the chaotic lifestyles sometimes observed in intravenous drug users means that the contraceptive needs of such women need careful thought and discussion.

The combined oral contraceptive pill is more likely to be contra-indicated, barrier methods of contraception are less likely to be religiously used, the intra-uterine contraceptive device may be less widely advocated in a group at increased risk of pelvic sepsis anyway and the progesterone-only pill may have an unacceptably high failure rate. Injectable methods of contraception (such as depot medroxy-progesterone acetate) have much to offer in that they are in general believed to be non-toxic to the liver, have a negligible failure rate providing that they are given when due, are convenient in that they are non-intercourse related and do not require a daily 'routine'. However, there is at least a theoretical risk that they may induce or aggravate osteoporosis in those patients who already are, or may become, amenorrhoeic as a result of progesterone injections.

Osteoporosis and amenorrhoea

Osteoporosis, secondary to prolonged amenorrhoea, occurs as a result of low oestrogen levels and is more likely in women whose amenorrhoea is of greater than five years duration, who are significantly underweight and who are cigarette smokers. Measurement of plasma oestradiol level (values < 100 pmol/l indicates an increased risk of osteoporosis), bone density studies or the administration of a progestogen challenge test (5 mg of oral medroxyprogesterone acetate daily for five days will produce a 'withdrawal bleed' if the patient's oestrogen levels are normal) can help to establish those patients at significant risk of osteoporosis.[12]

Investigating the intravenous drug user

Baseline investigations (see Table 3.1) are particularly useful in the assessment of an intravenous drug user's health. Such tests can provide much information that is an invaluable aid to the interpretation of a sometimes vague history, multiple symptomatology and non-specific signs with which substance misusers may present. In addition, unsuspected disease can be identified and susceptibility to preventable diseases (such as hepatitis A and B) can be determined.

The screening of urine for drugs of abuse can provide verification of which drugs are used and can be a useful tool in the assessment of a drug user's treatment progress. Routine 'dip-stick' testing of urine for blood, protein, glucose and the presence of leukocytes may furnish evidence of previously unsuspected renal disease or diabetes and may provide confirmatory evidence of suspected urinary tract infection.

Blood tests can be difficult to perform on intravenous drug users with extensively damaged peripheral veins. Inspection of sites such as the posterior of the forearm (less accessible to those self-injecting and therefore commonly preserved), the back of the hands and the dorsum of the feet can demonstrate the presence of patent veins. Some intravenous drug users may offer to take their own blood samples, particularly those who are aware that they have poor venous access and who regularly inject themselves into the femoral veins.

A simple full blood count not uncommonly reveals unsuspected but significant anaemia (often due to iron deficiency) and the mean corpuscular volume is frequently raised in patients misusing alcohol. A white cell count and differential are useful in the diagnosis of acute infections. Liver function tests are often abnormal in intravenous drug users largely due to the prevalence of hepatitis B and C in this population and the high incidence of alcoholism. Abnormally raised liver enzymes may often provide the first indication of an otherwise 'silent', but acute, infection with hepatitis B.

Hepatitis B

Serological testing for hepatitis B markers will identify which patients have previously been exposed to the disease, which remain carriers and which should be offered hepatitis B vaccine. Hepatitis B remains prevalent amongst intravenous drug users and up to half of those screened show evidence of previous infection,[13] although many can recall no episode of jaundice. The disease is particularly virulent in drug users because there is often concomitant infection with hepatitis D.[14] Few intravenous drug users show evidence of previous vaccination against hepatitis B despite the fact that vaccine has been available since 1981 and they are at high risk of contracting the illness.[15] This may reflect the limited availability of both screening and vaccination in drug treatment clinics,[16] the difficulty that some drug users experience registering with a GP, and the fact that there is some evidence suggesting that intravenous drug users may not mount as effective an immune response when vaccine is administered.[17] Hepatitis B is likely to remain an important cause of mortality and morbidity in substance misusers until effective vaccination rates are achieved. Vaccination also provides protection against hepatitis D.

If any group of professionals can begin to break the chain of hepatitis B infection in intravenous drug users then hope must lie with GPs. Vaccines available are safe, have few reported side-effects, and can (and should) be given to those who are HIV positive and are not contraindicated in pregnancy. Post-vaccination serology is needed to determine whether immunity has been successfully conferred. Several booster doses may be needed to achieve adequate seroconversion.

Hepatitis C

Serological testing for hepatitis C antibodies requires careful counselling of the patient before it is undertaken. Evidence of hepatitis C infection is found in 50–70% of intravenous drug users in the developed world and effective treatments are neither fully developed nor universally available. Unlike infection with the hepatitis B virus most patients with hepatitis C appear to remain carriers. Modes of transmission are less clearly ascertained than for hepatitis B but it is understood that the sharing of needles and injecting equipment is an important factor in the spread of this virus in the drug-using population. It is anticipated that a significant number of those suffering from hepatitis C will develop progressive liver disease[18] but there are no reliable indicators to determine which of those infected with hepatitis C will do so and most studies have been conducted on non drug users who contracted the disease from blood transfusions. Some patients prefer not to know their hepatitis C status. Others, accepting that they are likely to harbour the virus anyway, choose to be tested. A positive test for hepatitis C antibodies can inspire drug users susceptible to hepatitis B infection to ensure that they are vaccinated, may influence some to modify their alcohol and drug abuse and can enable monitoring and available treatment to be offered to those known to be infected. Many patients with hepatitis C are asymptomatic and few report jaundice. Others experience a variety of symptoms, including vague malaise, fatigue, abdominal discomfort, nausea and anorexia.

HIV

HIV testing may be requested by intravenous drug users who perceive themselves to be at risk of having contracted the virus. The incidence of positive HIV tests in injecting drug users varies across the UK. Data from the unlinked anonymous HIV prevalence programme for 1993 gave prevalence figures of 4% and 2.8% for male and female drug users respectively living in London and the South East, and 0.6% for men and 0.7% for women living elsewhere.[19] A recent audit of HIV-test requests in a large London teaching hospital found that 16% of intravenous drug users tested proved to be HIV positive, raising the worrying possibility that prevalence surveys may be underestimating the true rate of infection.[20] Nevertheless, figures in the UK are relatively low in comparison to some other European countries, particularly Italy, France, Spain and Switzerland. This has importance because travel between European countries is now widespread and the relative availability of methadone treatment in the UK means that a significant number of other European intravenous drug users seek help with their drug dependency here. HIV tests performed on intravenous drug users from other European countries with a higher prevalence of HIV amongst the drug using population are more likely to be positive.

It is important that issues such as the likelihood of a positive test result, the potential social and financial implications of a positive result, the patient's understanding of what a positive test means medically and what supports are available to him or her are discussed and documented before testing is undertaken. Many drug users are unclear about the difference between an HIV test and a diagnosis of AIDS, others may ask for an HIV test hoping to be reassured by a negative result without having fully contemplated the possibility that the test could be positive. Sometimes, an HIV test is required immediately after an episode of high-risk behaviour such as needle-sharing and the patient then needs to be advised that testing may not provide a reliable result until sufficient time has elapsed for the development of antibodies. A wait of three months between the last episode of risk-taking and the performing of the test is advisable and provides an accurate result in 99% of cases. Once an HIV test has been taken, advising of a definite date by which the result will be available can both spare the patient the anxiety of an indeterminate wait and allow the GP a planned consultation in which to give the result. HIV-test results should ideally be given by the person who organized the test, and in person. Post-test counselling can be undertaken at the time a result is given and for those who test negative can involve useful discussion about safer drug use or sexual behaviour. Patients testing positive will need clear advice about onward medical referral, some may request confirmatory testing and all will need emotional support. Post-test counselling of the newly diagnosed HIV-positive patient is rarely confined to one circumscribed session in which the result is given, and may usefully involve other health professionals and other agencies.

Summary

Ill health amongst substance misusers produces much misery for the individuals themselves and constitutes an important threat to public health as the number of drug abusers continues to rise. The cost of providing acute or emergency treatment for illnesses that could have been prevented, or at least detected at an earlier stage, continues to be high. By virtue of their broad training and experience, and because of their accessibility, GPs are in a unique position to meet the diverse needs of drug users. Many of the perceived negative aspects of treating a population of patients whose chemical dependency often remains a relapsing problem can be greatly diminished if GPs can also focus on providing general medical care to a patient group who, whilst challenging, can also be stimulating, interesting and rewarding. Few other patients provide so many real opportunities to prevent, detect and treat significant diseases and few are more in need of the services that a GP can provide.

4

Counselling drug users

Brian Whitehead

Counselling is an important adjunct to the helping process when working with drug users. Fortunate GPs will have access to specialist counselling services for drug users, but all GPs can and should understand what counselling is aiming to do, and its role in the care of drug users. This chapter explores the process of counselling and describes some techniques to assist GPs in their work with drug users.

Counselling aims to assist clients in making changes to their lives. Counselling in general practice offers the opportunity to support drug users through the change process and to assist them in achieving the goals that they have identified. It supports and parallels other aspects of treatment that are negotiated between GP and patient.

General practitioners are likely to be consulted by a wide variety of drug users. They should be able to respond to the needs of users who present across the range of experimental, recreational, social, dependent and long-term use. It is recognized that brief interventions can effect change even in those who perceive few problems with their drug use and that change can also be effected with long-term poly-drug users who are likely to present with a wider range of psycho-social problems.

Facilitating change

Assessing a client's motivation to change is a central component in the assessment and treatment process. When working with drug users it is necessary to establish what goals they want to achieve and what changes they wish to effect, both in their drug use and in other aspects of their lives. It is important to establish mutually agreed and realistic goals that can be achieved. Some points to bear in mind are listed below.

- In order to change, people must be motivated for and believe that the change will do some good, and believe that they have a reasonable chance of achieving it.

- People engage in behaviours that are meaningful and purposeful to them. Attempts should be made to understand the motivation for engaging in behaviours despite the adverse consequences.

- Change should be consistent with the individual's beliefs, values and behaviour.

- People need assistance and support in order to change and will not be completely successful in adhering to all new behaviours.

- It is often easier to get people to modify a behaviour than to eliminate it.

- Incremental behaviour change is important to recognize. Global lifestyle changes come slowly, and build upon previous successes.

- Instead of looking at what has to change, look at what can remain the same.

Stages of change

It is generally recognized that drug use is a chronic, relapsing condition. It is therefore important to be able to recognize where a client may be in this process so that interventions can be targeted most appropriately. A helpful model for understanding the processes that a drug user may move through is the Cycle or Stages of Change Model developed by Prochaska and Di Clemente (Figure 4.1).[1]

This model describes a six-phase cycle of change that helps to explain how people change. There are a series of stages through which people pass in the course of a problem. It also assists GPs in being able to assess drug users to determine which interventions would be most appropriate at a particular time in their progress through their change.

The model is described as a wheel, which reflects that in almost any change it is normal for the person to go round the process several times before achieving a stable change. Prochaska and Di Clemente in their original research with smokers found that clients ordinarily progressed through the cycle between three and seven times before finally quitting for good. This model recognizes that relapse is a normal occurrence or stage of change. By assessing these separate and different stages of readiness to change the model suggests that different approaches, strategies and interventions can be used depending on where the user is in the process of change. Different skills will be

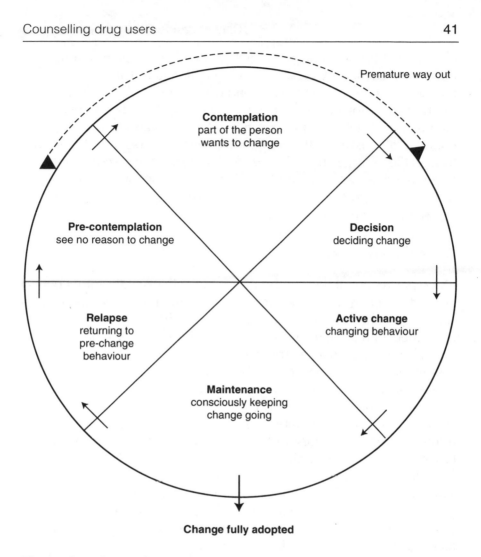

Figure 4.1: Cycle of change

needed in working with a user in the contemplation stage rather than in the action stage. Indeed, the model proposes that problems of client resistance or of being unmotivated occur when the worker is using strategies inappropriate for a client's current stage of change.

Pre-contemplation

The entry point to the process of change is the *pre-contemplation stage*. Often at this point the user has not even considered the possibility of change, not having contemplated there being a problem or a need to make any change. A person who is challenged at this stage about having a problem is likely to respond with surprise. Pre-contemplators rarely present for treatment *per se*. They may have been coerced to attend and are likely to present in a defensive manner. The term pre-contemplator assumes that someone else recognizes a problem even though the user may not self-identify. Clients in the pre-contemplation stage need information and feedback to raise awareness of the problem and possibility of change. Providing prescriptive advice at this stage can be unhelpful and counterproductive.

Contemplation and decision

Once awareness of their problems occurs, clients enter into a period characterized by ambivalence and attachment: the *contemplation stage*. This phase is characterized by a double-sided ambivalence; to change, to remain the same. The user at this time will be considering and rejecting change. The experience can best be described as a seesaw between reasons to stay the same and reasons to change. The contemplator simultaneously experiences reasons for concern, and motivations for change and to continue unchanged. The task at this stage is to explore the ambivalence and attachment to present and future desired behaviours and to tip the balance in favour of change. Once clients have examined and explored their ambivalence they may decide to change or not to change. They will then move into a stage of *decision*. This provides a window of opportunity to reflect on the advantages and disadvantages of change and to assist the user to consider what and how they are considering changing. The GP can facilitate the user to consider and identify which change strategy is acceptable, accessible, appropriate and effective.

Action and maintenance

The action phase then facilitates the first steps towards the client's action plan. Here the client engages in specific actions to bring about change. These efforts may or may not require the use of formal counselling. The goal during this phase is to assist and facilitate a change in the problem area. However, initiating change is only the beginning of the change process, not the end. The maintenance phase is characterized not by an absence of change but maintenance of it. Making a change does not guarantee that the change will be maintained. It is accepted that in some change strategies there may be lapses (slips) or a return to pre-change behaviour (relapse). During this phase the goal is to support the change brought about by action, and to prevent relapse. Maintaining a change requires a different set of skills and techniques to those needed initially to achieve the change. Being abstinent, stabilizing, maintenance, harm minimization, risk reduction, reduced offending and many of the other change behaviours desired in the drug user are the initial action steps followed by the challenge of maintaining the behaviour. Slips and relapses are normal and expected occurrences as a user works to change long-established behaviour patterns. The task is to support the user to contemplate change, support change already begun and to resume action strategies.

Interventions according to the Cycle of Change

Stages of change	GP task
Pre-contemplation	Increase the user's perception of risk and problems with present behaviour
Contemplation	Identify attachment to behaviours. Explore ambivalence Elicit reasons to change, costs of staying the same Tip the balance. Emphasis on client's desired change Support client's self-esteem and competence for change
Decision	Explore with the user the best course of action to take in change, strategies and interventions
Action	Help the client to take steps towards change
Maintenance	Identify and use strategies to maintain and support change
Relapse	Facilitate progress through the stages of change. Support the client once again passing through contemplation, decision and action

Motivating clients

Motivating clients is a central and essential part of a GP's role. The ability to adhere to a programme of change is associated with successful outcomes. Motivation can be defined as 'the probability that a person will enter into, continue, and adhere to a specific change strategy'. It is the GP's responsibility not only to provide advice but to motivate, and to increase the likelihood that the client will follow a desired course of action towards change. Users may be motivated to engage or participate in one form of treatment but not another, to work on one problem but not another, or to continue to see one worker but not another. A user may not want detoxification but may be motivated to reduce harm or stabilize drug use. This specificity is all too readily confirmed by clinical experience and further clarifies that motivation is not a general 'have' or 'have not' trait of the individual but depends on the context.

Motivational strategies

What strategies can be used by the GP to enhance motivation for change? If motivation is a behavioural probability what strategies or techniques can be used that increase the probability of change? Research shows that most people who change their addictive behaviour do so without ever entering formal treatment. Most people who have problems with alcohol, smoking or illicit drugs resolve or reduce their problems without the intervention of professionals. Many patients report that they achieved this change by deciding to change, triggered by either an internal or external cue, but experienced as an internalized process of decision making, and by embracing a commitment to change. This internal process of decision making and commitment is a central and essential element in effecting change. It is often easier within the time-limited constraints of general practice to focus on the 'how' of changing without giving considered attention to the decision and commitment to change. This may be detrimental and counterproductive. General practitioners need to understand that in work with patients who present with problems requiring change, it is more important to clarify decisions and build commitment to change than to focus primarily on initiating change. Once this motivational decision has been reached, processes and strategies can then be targeted to assist clients to identify their own resources for effecting change.

Brief interventions

Brief interventions have developed from the belief that change is essentially motivational, and that with examination of commitment to change, and clarification of the decisions to change, clients can apply their own natural ability to effect change. Brief interventions demonstrate better results than if clients receive no counselling, and appear to have comparable results to longer-term interventions.[2]

The components of a brief intervention strategy have been summarized by the acronym FRAMES:

- feedback
- responsibility
- advice
- menu
- empathy
- self-efficacy.

1 Feedback

Feedback typically includes a structured and comprehensive assessment, through which the client is given feedback. This provides clients with an objective picture of their situation and allows for reflection on problem areas in their lives.

2 Responsibility

Great emphasis is placed on the responsibility of the client to effect change. The GP is only a supporter of any change that the client determines is of importance. This often needs to be made explicit. Implicit in the process of the client taking responsibility is for the GP to provide self-assessment and self-help guides, for clear process assessment and change planning.

3 Advice

Advice should be based on an objective assessment of the client. Accurate and non-judgemental information can be given to clients to assist them to draw their own conclusions from the facts, based upon assessment. The GP is in an important position to provide such information to the patients.

4 Menu

Clients are more likely to effect and maintain change if they perceive the benefit of change and then identify the most appropriate strategies to achieve this. Clients should be offered a list (menu) of optional strategies to consider. Prescribing a single-change strategy is unlikely to be as effective as the option of choice. Choice gives clients the opportunity to select approaches that meet their particular needs and situation. Empowering users with the freedom to select strategies also enhances personal control, and if they perceive that they chose a particular course of action they are more likely to persist and maintain any change effect.

Clarifying what is available also allows GPs to reflect upon and define the boundaries and limits of their practice. It then becomes evident what is required in terms of support from external agencies.

5 Empathy

The ability of a GP to express empathy is a well-recognized cornerstone of therapeutic relationship. The importance of the interpersonal relationship between users and their GPs should not be underestimated. Users who feel they are being judged and unwanted are more likely to be resistant to, and drop-out of, treatment.

6 Self-efficacy or competence

Users must be able to ascribe change to themselves, and be able to identify with the belief that they can change. Sustaining clients' belief in themselves is crucial for effecting change.

These six elements are the building blocks of any intervention. Together with the core principles of motivational interviewing[3] they create the environment in which the examination of attachment and ambivalence can begin.

Principles of motivational interviewing

- Express empathy
- Develop discrepancy
- Avoid argumentation
- Roll with resistance
- Support self-efficacy

Ambivalence is a normal state experienced in any change, and it is important to make use of this ambivalence within the client. Making clients aware of the consequences of their behaviour, whilst developing discrepancy between present behaviour and future desired goals, is the central element of any helping process.

A person contemplating change experiences competing motivations because there are both benefits and costs associated with both sides of the conflict. In the contemplation stage, a person is weighing up both the benefits and costs of change against the merits of continuing as before. There exists a motivational balance between staying the same and changing. The strategy for working with clients is to remove the emphasis on staying the same, and to focus on the change side of the scale. A helpful way of drawing out a specific problem with ambivalent clients is to elicit both sides of the coin, and to engage with clients in a cost–benefit analysis of their behaviour. This examines the perceived benefits of a behaviour against the perceived costs or disadvantages of an alternative course of action.

Cost–benefit analysis

Continue as before		*Make a change*	
Benefits	Costs	Benefits	Costs

A cost–benefit analysis draws attention to the discrepancy between present behaviour and broader goals – where a person is, as opposed to where they want to be. Users are often caught in this conflict between being attracted to, and repelled by, their behaviour. A GP's goal of motivating clients is to develop this discrepancy and amplify it until it overrides a client's attachment to their present behaviour.

A counselling framework for general practice

1 Establish therapeutic relationship

- Support self-esteem
- Support client competence (efficacy)
- Define boundaries
- Leave responsibility for change with client:
  - assess according to Stages of Change
  - why has client come to you?
  - what concerns does the client have?
  - what do they want to change? Why?
  - what do they want to keep the same?

2 What are the client's perceptions of the problem?

- What are your perceptions of the problem?
- Provide feedback: objective, factual, non-judgemental

3 History

- Gather psychological/social and other factors for motivation for change/staying the same
- Provide feedback

4 Goals

- What goals do they have? Match GPs agenda?
- Conduct cost–benefit analysis
- Identify sources of motivation for engaging in behaviour

5 Analysis of goal setting – specific, achievable (realistic), measurable?

- Construct hierarchy for goal achievement
  (Ladder 1–5, where 1 most achievable and 5 most difficult goal)
- Identify strategies to achieve goals
- Explore conflicts between goals
- Identify unrealistic goals
- Identify and explore rewards for goal achievement

5

Opiate misuse

Edwin Martin

Introduction

The definition of drug use as 'misuse' depends on what society will or will not tolerate, rather than on any logical assessment of risk and benefit. In the nineteenth century, opium and its derivatives were fashionable and popular drugs consumed everywhere from Fenland pubs to the salons of literary London.[1] Today, the use of opiate drugs, notably heroin, inspires passionate moral censure and attracts severe legal penalties.[2] In the Western world, attitudes to opiate users vary from tolerance and respect, with an offer of help in the Netherlands, to zero tolerance policies in the USA where drug use is strictly punished by law.[3] Medical involvement in opiate misuse in the UK has varied widely over the past 35 years. In the 1960s many doctors prescribed opiates to addicted patients and this was accepted practice. In the 1970s the view was that GPs should not prescribe opiates to these patients. In the 1980s government guidelines encouraged GPs to prescribe opiates on a reducing schedule for patients who had a habit, but not to prescribe maintenance doses.[4] In the 1990s, after HIV was recognized to be a major problem among drug users, GPs were advised to prescribe maintenance doses of oral opiates, but not to prescribe injectables.[5]

Opiate use today

The majority of drug users start experimenting with drugs in their teens or early adult life. At least part of this behaviour can be explained on the basis of adolescent rebellion and normal risk-taking behaviour. When the drug used is alcohol or tobacco, society takes a tolerant view of this behaviour. There is an expectation that those involved will grow out of the behaviour. Where the drug involved is cannabis or heroin, however, the behaviour is criminalized. Problems arise from this process of criminalization. First, it is estimated that in many areas of the UK nearly half of all young people in their middle teens will have used illegal drugs.[6] There is clearly a problem with criminalizing half of society's young people. If society wishes to stop young people using certain drugs, the criminal law may not be the best tool. Second, where there is a widespread market for any commodity, but the commodity cannot be acquired legally, the market will pass into the hands of the criminal underworld. The profits will be used to fund a wide variety of criminal activities.

Level of alcohol use during adolescence is a poor predictor of problem alcohol consumption in young adulthood.[7] Pandina and Schuele have argued for similarities with drug use.[8] It seems likely that young people do often 'grow out' of drug use. Many people seem able to discontinue opiate use without much difficulty. Those that become long-term opiate users may be people with more problems. Many of them have histories of physical and sexual abuse as children.[9] There tend to be larger numbers of opiate users in areas of poverty and where there is high unemployment.[2]

As with any illicit drug use, exact figures for prevalence are not available. Annual notifications to the Home Office by doctors in the UK report only those users who reveal their use to a doctor, and doctors may forget to notify. The Addicts Index recorded around 36 000 notifications of opiate use in 1995, compared with about 12 000 in 1988.[10] Just under half of those first notified in 1995 were aged under 25 and about three-quarters of them male. The Addicts Index was discontinued on 1 May 1997 and information on opiate use will no longer be available from that source. Additional information is available from the Drug Misuse Statistics Bulletin[11] that publishes information on a six-monthly basis obtained from regional drugs misuse databases to which any professional in contact with illicit drug users can notify. Figures for the six months March to September 1995 for England reported 22 848 users, of whom 21 555 were using opiates as a main or subsidiary drug (64% heroin, 30% methadone and 6% 'other opiates'). Almost half of the 15 822 reporting opiates as their main drug of use were injecting. These figures underestimate the true extent of use as they only represent clients newly presenting to the reporting agency during that time period, and obviously exclude opiate users who are not in contact with services. Clearly opiate misuse is a large and growing problem.

- In the nineteenth century opium derivatives were popular and widely used drugs. Today their use inspires passionate moral censure and severe legal penalties

- Attitudes to drug users vary from tolerance and the offer of help in the Netherlands to zero tolerance and strict punishment by law in the USA

- 75% of teenagers have been offered illegal drugs and 47% have tried them; 1–2% of the adult population uses illegal drugs

- It is estimated conservatively that 100 000 drug users in the UK each need to find £10 000 per year to fund their habit

- Notification to the Home Office of drug users increased by 80% between 1991 and 1995

- Drug users have a largely undeserved reputation for violence

- 40% of drug users may be able to abandon their habit with competent care in general practice

How opiates are used

People take opiates by a variety of routes. They may be taken orally, as mixtures, tablets or powders mixed with other agents. They may be inhaled either by heating over a flame on tin foil and inhaling the vapour, or in cigarette form. They may also be taken intravenously either using ampoules or dissolving opiate powder or crushed tablets. Since the rise in concern over the spread of HIV by sharing needles, this route is used less than previously. Less frequently the opiate may be taken as a suppository.

The most sought-after drug is heroin, though many other drugs such as Diconal, dihydrocodeine or pethidine are used. The effect of heroin is a feeling of alertness, followed by a feeling of warmth and contentment combined with drowsiness. If the drug is used intravenously it gives a distinctive 'buzz' within 1–2 minutes, which has been likened to an orgasm.[12] The drug may be obtained by theft from a chemist's shop, by diversion of prescribed drugs on to the street market, or by buying it (often cut with other substances) from a drug dealer. The drug market often functions in a pyramid fashion. Users sell some of their supplies on at a profit to fund their own habit. The people who make large profits from the sale of drugs may be several steps removed from the street scene and may not be drug users themselves.

A typical drug user's day

A long-term addicted opiate user may wake up in the morning already suffering from drug withdrawal symptoms. Many would have no food in the house at this time. They have to get up and shoplift or steal enough goods in other ways to be able to pay for their fixes that day. Having acquired the goods, they then have to find a 'fence' who will pay them about 10% of the value of the goods that they have stolen. Thus, to buy £80 worth of drugs (about 1 g) they would have to steal goods worth about £800. It has been estimated very conservatively that in the UK there are 100 000 opiate users each needing to raise £10 000 per year to fund their habit.[13] Having got their money, opiate users would then find their dealer and buy their drug supply for the day. The drug has a varying degree of purity and might contain different amounts of other substances – some of them toxic. If the drug user used the intravenous route and had clean needles and syringes, these would be used. However, if the needle exchange was some way away or closed, the user might share needles and syringes, perhaps after washing them out with soap and water. There is in some drug cultures an odd sense of fellowship involved in sharing equipment.[12] This habit has persisted despite people knowing the risks of catching HIV and hepatitis. After taking their drug, if users have any money left over, they might buy food or alcohol.

Health consequences of opiate use

Heroin users have a high risk of premature death, with death rates of 1–3%, the majority from overdose. Ill health associated with opiate misuse mainly results from the route of administration of the drug, particularly injecting, and the poor social conditions in which many users live. These health problems are described in other chapters and will not be discussed in detail here apart from overdose and withdrawals.

Overdose

Injecting opiate users are at risk from overdose. This may occur because of the varying purity of the drugs bought on the street. If an opiate user injects an unusually pure fix of heroin, he may overdose. Other situations where users may run into trouble with overdose are when they have temporarily lost their tolerance through being in prison or from having stopped using drugs for a while. If they start using opiates again and immediately take their previous dose they may die from overdose. Other patients run into problems combining prescribed or street opiates and depressant drugs like alcohol or benzodiazapines.

Opiate overdose leads to pinpoint pupils, varying degrees and depth of coma depending on the extent of the overdose, and respiratory depression. Patients may vomit and inhale the vomit.

Treatment

The specific antidote is naloxone. GPs should consider carrying naloxone as an emergency drug.

- Give naloxone 400 mcg (1 amp) intravenously (IV), which should act within two minutes and 400 mcg intramuscularly (IM), which has a less rapid onset of action.
- If no, or only slight improvement, repeat with double the dose.
- If still no improvement, double the dose again and repeat.
- If there is still no response, the diagnosis of opiate overdose should be questioned.

Naloxone is short acting, and repeated injections may need to be given if a longer acting opiate, such as methadone has been taken. An ambulance should be called and the patient admitted to hospital.

Withdrawal syndromes

Withdrawal syndromes differ according to the particular form of opiate used, the daily amounts taken, the duration of use and individual sensitivity. Although very unpleasant, withdrawal is not life threatening. Users withdrawing from opiates may experience the following.

• Nausea, vomiting, diarrhoea.

• Restlessness, anxiety, irritability, sleeplessness.

• Pains in muscles, bones and joints.

• Running nose and eyes, sneezing, yawning, sweating.

• Dilated pupils.

• Gooseflesh, flushing.

It can be difficult to distinguish between symptoms of opiate and benzodiazepine withdrawals in polydrug users. The most reliable sign of opiate withdrawal is dilated pupils.

Treatment

If the patient is obviously suffering withdrawal symptoms, one or more of the following drugs may be helpful in reducing the symptoms.

• *Lofexidine* – is related to clonidine but has less hypotensive action. It reduces symptoms such as sweats, diarrhoea and abdominal cramps but has no effect on bone and muscle pain, insomnia or craving for opiates. Designed for in-patient use, it can be used in small doses in general practice. Prescribe lofexidine 0.2 mg, one or two to be taken every six hours up to a maximum of six daily. Do not prescribe for more than a few days.

• *Diphenoxylate and atropine (Lomotil)* – a mild opioid with low addictive potential, helpful in management of diarrhoea. Give one tab stat, then two tabs six-hourly.

• *Mebeverine* – this can be used to reduce abdominal pain, cramps and diarrhoea. Use 135 mg t.d.s.

• *Thioridazine* – this is a phenothiazine tranquillizer with virtually no addictive potential. It may reduce the agitation or insomnia associated with opiate withdrawal. Dosage is 25 mg t.d.s. or 50–100 mg nocte.

Care of opiate users in general practice

The view of drug users held by GPs has been found to closely approximate that held by middle-class people in general. Users are categorized as violent, deceitful and disruptive.[14,15] In reality, opiate users usually only act in a criminal fashion in the context of obtaining resources to fund their drug habit. In a stable therapeutic relationship they are rarely violent.[16] Opiate users are unwelcome in many practices.[17] Many GPs will not register users and will strike them off their lists as soon as their addiction becomes apparent.[18]

Principles of managing drug use

- In a democracy a GP cannot and does not have the right to make anybody do anything

- A GP cannot make a person stop taking a substance that is freely, though illegally, available for sale on the street simply by telling him or her to stop, or by prescribing a reducing dose of this class of substance

- If GPs want to help patients, they must start where the patients are and address the patients' agenda, rather than starting where they themselves would like the patients to be and trying to get the patients to address the GP's agenda

---

The minimal service that a GP should afford to opiate users is care of their general health and referral to the local drug service for management of their drug problems. However, general practice is the ideal place for management of all of a drug user's problems, including prescribing replacement drugs. Competent care for opiate users has been shown to reduce their mortality eight-fold.[19] Methadone prescribing is addressed in more detail in Chapter 6. The advantage of providing a full range of care for patients within the practice is that their opiate habit is dealt with alongside the usual medical problems about which people consult their GP, and the patient is not stigmatized. Opiate users also prefer to receive their care from GPs.[20]

Engaging with opiate users is worthwhile. Our practice in Bedfordshire found that 40% of the 155 patients cared for who were using opiates over a ten-year period stopped taking drugs.[21] There were patients of all ages and all degrees of motivation. When an opiate user was accepted on to the practice list the only contract made was that he or she should not carry out any violent act toward the GP, the staff, other patients or the practice building.

The six aims of the care of opiate users in our programme were as follows.

1   To give patients personal space and allow their days to be less fraught and more structured.

2   To form a trusting, non-judgemental relationship with them.

3   To help them look at how they got into the situation they were in.

4   To encourage them to consider whether they were happy with their present situation.

5   To consider ways they would like to change their lives.

6   To consider precisely what they wanted to do about changing their situation and what resources they needed to help them do this.

As part of giving these patients space, methadone was prescribed for them by their normal administration route. A dedicated drug support worker was employed by the practice with funding from the health authority. A three-way meeting between the doctor, the patient and the drug worker took place every three months. This was in addition to the usual consultations between GP and patient, and between the patient and the drug support worker. During these meetings no pressure was put on the patient to reduce his or her dose of drug or to stop injecting.

Topics of discussion usually centred around matters such as housing, nutrition, personal problems and what plans, if any, the patient had for his or her life. The patient set the agenda and the GP and drug support worker worked with the patient by generating priorities. Patients at times planned changes to their lives and then did not succeed in carrying out these plans. However, it was accepted that drug misuse is a chronic, relapsing condition. The patient was not rejected, but his or her agenda was redefined and priorities addressed. Outcome measures such as a decrease in criminal activities, getting back together with a partner, getting children back from care and obtaining secure housing or a job were counted as just as important as any change in opiate use.

The disadvantage of providing this kind of service is that care of these people takes an enormous amount of a GP's time. I have estimated that they need up to twenty times as much time as non drug-using patients. Also, once it becomes known that a practice gives effective care to drug users, word gets around the drug-using community and there could be demand from other opiate users to register. Practices may find they have to limit the number of drug users they care for. Nevertheless, the rewards for the patient and the GP outweigh these disadvantages. It is to be hoped that increasing numbers of practices will become involved in caring for this group of patients. This will ease the pressures on those GPs currently trying to meet the demand for care from opiate users and enable many more drug users to benefit from the effective help available to them from general practice.

6

Methadone prescribing

Judy Bury

The prescribing of methadone as a substitute drug is now an accepted part of the management of opiate users and has many potential benefits.[1-3] It reduces the risk of opiate injecting and of needle sharing and the need for criminal activity to buy street drugs. By providing a regular supply of medication and reducing withdrawal symptoms, it offers opiate users an opportunity to stabilize their drug intake and their lifestyle. Prescribing also helps to keep drug users in contact with health services with the potential for offering physical health care and counselling

---

Benefits of methadone prescribing for opiate users

- Reduces risk of injecting and needle sharing

- Reduces need for criminal activity to buy street drugs

- Reduces or prevents withdrawal symptoms

- Offers opportunity to stabilize drug intake and lifestyle

- Helps to keep drug user in contact with health services

Many GPs are reluctant to prescribe methadone. They fear attracting too many drug users to their surgery, are concerned that these sometimes difficult patients may upset their staff or other patients, and may also be concerned that the methadone they prescribe may be sold.[4,5] With appropriate precautions, it is possible to limit the diversion of prescribed methadone.[5] If drug users are managed in a firm but considerate manner, with the use of clear agreements and consistent boundaries, the work can be satisfying and rewarding, with minimal disruption to the practice and with both physical and emotional benefits for the drug user.[5]

Why methadone?

Many drugs have been used as substitute medication for opiate users, for example dihydrocodeine and buprenorphine. The main advantages of methadone are that the mixture is less likely to be injected and it is longer acting than other opiates. If given in the right dose it can prevent withdrawal symptoms for 24 hours and usually without giving any stimulant effect or 'buzz' after it is taken. This can help drug users to achieve some stability in their lives, which then allows other problems to be tackled. Its long duration of action means that it is easy to titrate to get the dose correct and it is practical to supervise its consumption. The other advantages of methadone are that it is less likely to be sold than shorter acting tablets that are more easily transportable and that give more 'buzz', and that its use has been well researched.[1-3] The main disadvantage of methadone is that its long duration of action makes it more dangerous in overdose, especially if taken with other CNS depressants, including alcohol.

   Methadone is a remarkably safe drug when used long term and side-effects are relatively infrequent. They include respiratory depression, constipation, sweating, dental decay and weight gain, the last two due in part to the sugar content of the usual formulation (methadone mixture).

Prescribing in general practice or by a specialist service?

There has been much debate about the appropriate setting for methadone prescribing. The experience from a number of areas suggests that this work can be done successfully in general practice,[6,7] particularly if GPs have had training and have the support of a specialist agency.[8] When GPs first become involved in this work, they may wish all their drug users to be assessed by the agency. In areas where a shared-care model has developed, the agency then recommends to the GP what to prescribe and offers counselling and support to the drug user, while the GP issues the prescription and provides physical care for the drug user.[8] In some areas, staff from a drug agency will see drug users on surgery premises and discuss cases periodically with GPs on site.

As GPs become more familiar with the issues and build up confidence in this area of work, they may feel able to assess the drug user and initiate a prescription themselves, knowing that advice and support from the drug agency is available. If problems arise, the drug user can be referred for further assessment or, in the case of more difficult users, have their care taken over for a while by the specialist service.

When to start prescribing methadone

A prescription for methadone as a substitute opiate should only be considered if, after full assessment:

- opiates are present in the urine. (In exceptional circumstances a script may be started without waiting for a urine screen result, e.g. groin injecting, pregnancy with recent trackmarks, drug user is ill and withdrawing, post-prison with recent trackmarks (but start with low dose))

- opiates are being taken daily

- there is convincing evidence of dependence, including objective signs of withdrawal (e.g. dilated pupils)

- the drug user seems motivated to stabilize his or her drug use

- the GP and the drug user are clear that a substitute prescription could help to achieve certain goals.

Setting goals

Before prescribing any substitute drug it is important to establish what goals the GP and the drug user hope to achieve.

The doctor's goals

In prescribing methadone as a substitute opiate, the GP should be aiming to:

- find the level of methadone that prevents opiate withdrawal symptoms and reduces the need for the drug user to take additional illicit opiates

- support the drug user to achieve a level of stability where other issues can be tackled by the drug user, alone or with the support of the GP or other agencies

- keep the drug user in contact with the GP so that their health can be monitored.

The drug user's goals

It is important to establish with drug users what changes they wish to make to the way they use drugs and/or to other aspects of their life and in what way a substitute prescription might help them to achieve these changes. In the light of the changes that the drug user would like to make, it is then possible to set some mutually agreed and realistic goals to be achieved within three to four months of starting the substitute prescription. For example, drug users may wish to reduce and stop their drug injecting or to reduce and stop using drugs bought from the street. They may agree that they wish to be intoxicated less often or that they wish to improve relationships with their partner or parents.

It is important that the GP helps the drug user to set short-term goals that are realistic and achievable. For example, it is unrealistic to expect someone who has been using drugs for a long time to come off drugs quickly and stay off, or someone who has been unemployed for a long time to find employment within a few months. If the goals are unrealistic and drug users fail to achieve them, they will feel a failure and the GP will become disillusioned. On the other hand, if appropriate short-term goals are achieved, the confidence and self-esteem of the drug user may be boosted and the GP will feel that progress is being made.

Once the GP and the drug user have agreed on appropriate goals, these can be written in the notes and reassessed after a few months. If some progress has been achieved, new short-term goals can be agreed. If nothing has been achieved then the prescription may need to be reconsidered and/or the drug user may need to be referred for specialist advice.

If drug users are very chaotic when first seen, it may be necessary to establish them on a prescription before suitable goals can be discussed and agreed but it should still be made clear to the drug user that this is a short-term measure to reduce chaos. If the chaos does not lessen after a few weeks, the appropriateness of the prescription should be reconsidered.

Goals should be reviewed periodically while substitute medication is being described.

How to prescribe methadone

The aim is to prescribe the lowest dose of methadone that will prevent withdrawal symptoms, minimize injecting and reduce the need for additional street drugs. There is evidence that higher doses of methadone (60 mg and above) are more effective than lower doses in reducing the risk of continued use of illicit opiates.[1,2] As long as the GP can be confident that the user is not oversedated and is not selling the medication, then there is no advantage in keeping the dose down at a level that leaves the drug user feeling uncomfortable. It is important to remember that many opiate users experience psychological withdrawal symptoms before they experience physical withdrawal symptoms.

Calculating the starting dose

During assessment, the drug user should be asked to complete a daily drug diary from which the average daily intake of opiates can be assessed. In discussion with the user, it is usually possible to establish the level of opiates that will prevent withdrawal. Using a conversion table (see Table 6.1) the equivalent methadone dose can then be calculated. It is advisable to start a little lower than this as it is often possible to achieve stability on a lower dose of methadone and, if not, it is easy to increase the dose. In addition, there is always the risk that the drug user has been exaggerating his or her intake of drugs.

Example: Drug user claims to be taking 25–30 tablets of 30 mg dihydrocodeine per day. He acknowledges that 20 tablets per day would probably be sufficient to prevent withdrawal. The equivalent dose of methadone is 60 mg. Start on 40 mg and increase as necessary.

The process of calculating the starting dose is easier if the opiate user has been taking pharmaceutical drugs such as buprenorphine, dihydrocodeine, dipipanone or dextramoramide than if the user has been injecting or smoking street heroin. In the latter case the user can be started on a prescription for 40 mg methadone a day, which can subsequently be increased according to the response.

Table 6.1: Opiate/opioid equivalents

Drug	Dose	Equivalent methadone dose
Street heroin		Cannot be estimated accurately due to variations in purity of street drugs. Start at 40 mg and increase as required.
Pharmaceutical heroin	10 mg ampoule or tablet	20 mg
Pethidine	50 mg ampoule or tablet	5 mg
Morphine	10 mg ampoule or tablet	10 mg
Dipipanone (Diconal)	10 mg tablet	4 mg
Dextromoramide (Palfium)	5 mg tablet	5–10 mg
Buprenorphine (Temgesic)	200 µg orally	2.5 mg
	200 µg injected	5–10 mg
Dihydrocodeine	30 mg	3 mg
Codeine phosphate	15 mg tablet	1 mg
Codeine linctus	5 ml	1 mg

Although the assessment process should identify those who are not already dependent on and tolerant to opiates, this will not always be the case. To avoid the danger of overdose in an individual who is not already opiate tolerant, the starting dose of methadone should not exceed 50 mg, regardless of the amount the user claims to have been using. The dose can subsequently be increased until an adequate dose is reached.

Pharmacology of methadone

Once a patient is established on methadone, it has a half-life of between 13 and 47 hours (average 25 hours) but it takes about three days before a steady state is reached.[9] From the drug users' point of view this means that they may continue to experience withdrawal for the first few days until they are settled on the correct dose. From the prescribers' point of view, this means that it is not possible to judge whether the prescribed dose is correct until this steady state is reached – so if the starting dose is increased, this should be done slowly.

Methadone preparations

The most convenient preparation of methadone to use is methadone mixture 1 mg per ml. This is a green liquid containing methadone hydrochloride, colouring (tartrazine and Green S), glucose syrup and chloroform water. A sugar-free preparation of methadone is also now available. Methadone tablets should be avoided as they are more likely to be injected.

Writing a methadone prescription

Prescriptions for controlled drugs in Schedules 1, 2 and 3, which include methadone, must be written in ink and must be signed and dated by the GP. Everything on the prescription including the patient's name and address, the form and strength of the preparation, the dose to be taken and the quantity must be in the GP's own handwriting. If the prescription is to be dispensed in instalments, the prescription must also specify in the GP's handwriting the number of instalments, the quantity per instalment and the intervals to be observed. Further information and a specimen prescription are in the BNF.

Methadone prescriptions can be written on an ordinary FP10 (or GP10 in Scotland). However, if daily or interval dispensing is required, GPs in England and Wales should use the blue form FP10 (MDA). This allows interval dispensing from a single prescription for 14 days.

GPs who are prescribing for ten or more drug users may apply to the Home Office Drugs Branch for exemption from handwriting requirements.

Liaising with the pharmacist

It is important to agree with the patient which pharmacist they will attend and then contact the pharmacist to confirm that he or she is willing to dispense methadone for this patient and to confirm the dispensing arrangements. It is helpful to record the name and telephone number of the pharmacist in the notes.

Supervision consumption

It is advisable to arrange for methadone consumption to be super-vised for the first few days to ensure that the full dose is taken by the patient and is not diverted and to ensure that the dose in neither too high nor too low. Consumption can be supervised by a drug agency, in the surgery or on pharmacy premises.

- If a *local drug agency* is able to offer this service, most GPs prefer to refer patients to the agency to start them on methadone until they feel they have acquired the experience and confidence to do this themselves.

- If consumption is to be supervised *in the surgery*, give a pre-scription for one day's methadone to the patient and ask him or her to collect this from the pharmacy and return. The patient should be observed taking the medication and then reviewed after four to six hours when maximum blood levels will have been reached, to check that the patient is not intoxicated or drowsy. This check is only required after the first dose, or if the dose has been increased by more than 10 mg per day.

- If the GP wishes consumption of the methadone to be supervised *on pharmacy premises*, the pharmacist should be approached to ask if he or she is willing to do this. It should be specified on the prescription that supervision is requested ('Please supervise con-sumption') and the patient should be told that the daily dose is to be consumed in the pharmacy. The patient should be asked to return to the surgery four to six hours after the first dose of methadone to check that he or she is not intoxicated or drowsy.
  The pharmacist may be willing to supervise the consumption of methadone for a few days or for longer[9] in which case he or she may develop a set or rules to be explained to the patient at the outset, e.g. time of day to attend, behaviour to be expected in the pharmacy.[10] The pharmacist can be asked to withhold the daily dose and contact the prescribing GP if the patient is intoxicated or if his or her behaviour is unacceptable.

Titrating the dose of methadone

Methadone should usually be taken between 9 and 10 a.m. in a once-daily dose. Patients should be seen after two days of methadone before the third morning dose to see if they are withdrawn. If there is evidence of withdrawal, the methadone dose should be increased by 5–10 mg. This process can be repeated until a level of methadone is reached that holds the patient for 24 hours without significant withdrawal but does not make them drowsy.

Objective signs of opiate withdrawal include a rapid pulse, sweating and dilated pupils. Even if the methadone dose is insufficient, opiate users may feel well for some hours after taking the morning dose but will begin to feel withdrawn (sweaty, agitated) later in the day or during the night, thus affecting their sleep. The earlier they experience these symptoms, the more the dose needs to be increased. This can be done in steps and the dose should not be increased by more than 10 mg per day in one step without close supervision.

Many opiate users do better if they are on more than the minimum amount needed to prevent physical withdrawal. If users continue to feel uncomfortable on the prescribed dose or continues to use additional street opiates, the dose of methadone should be increased. This can be done safely as long as they are seen not to be drowsy four to six hours after the daily dose has been consumed under supervision.

Dispensing arrangements

Methadone should be dispensed daily until the drug user is settled on a satisfactory dose level. If consumption is to be supervised, then obviously methadone must continue to be dispensed daily. Otherwise the dispensing arrangements will depend on the stability of the drug user. At first users may be tempted to take more than their daily dose each day and daily dispensing will prevent them running out of medication before their next prescription is due. As they become more stable, the dispensing intervals can be increased to alternate days and then to twice weekly. Once very stable, they might manage one week's supply at a time but few can manage more than this. If their drug use becomes chaotic again – often first demonstrated by returning early for a prescription – it is usually supportive to return to daily dispensing, although this change will often be resisted.

Patient information

When giving a prescription for methadone, the GP should warn the drug user that, although the methadone is safe for them, it could be dangerous for anyone who is not opiate tolerant, so the user has a responsibility to keep their medication in a safe place.

The user should also be warned that, as a CNS depressant, methadone will have an additive effect with other drugs causing CNS depression including alcohol, benzodiazepines and tricyclic antidepressants.

It is also helpful to give the user written information about methadone. *The Methadone Handbook* is a useful publication obtainable from ISDD, Waterbridge House, 32–36 Loman Street, London SE1 0EE.

Review

Once patients are stable on methadone, it may not be necessary to see them to issue a prescription more frequently than monthly unless they are actively working on problems or want to reduce their medication. Dispensing arrangements should be decided independently of how frequently the user needs to be seen.

It is important to carry out a thorough review periodically to assess how the drug user is progressing. Every four to six months review:

- how the user is progressing

- what ongoing problems he or she still has, including extra drug use

- what has been achieved since the last review – goals can be reviewed and new goals set if appropriate

- the need for additional support and/or counselling.

It is particularly important to review the dose of methadone. If the user is buying extra drugs this may be because the prescribed dose is too low.

Urine toxicology

Checking the urine should be part of the review process but is best carried out randomly. Toxicology is usually carried out by clinical chemistry laboratories. The main purpose is to confirm that the methadone has been taken and to find out what other drugs have been taken.

The user should be asked to provide a specimen on the premises and the GP can then check that it is warm (and therefore likely to be the user's own). If methadone has been taken within the previous 24 hours, urine toxicology should be positive but administrative and laboratory errors do occur. However, if the urine repeatedly shows no methadone then it is likely that the user is not taking what is prescribed and the prescription should be stopped. With regard to other drugs, the main purpose of checking the urine is to encourage openness so that problems can be addressed, rather than to punish the user by reducing or stopping the prescription if other drug use is identified.

What action should be taken after a urine test result?

1   *Positive for methadone and opiate*: Discuss script with user. Why using drug on top? Dose of methadone inadequate? More pleasure from heroin?

2   *Positive for methadone/negative for opiates*: Using script only

3   *Negative for methadone/positive for opiates*: Selling methadone?

4   *Negative for methadone*: Switch to daily dispensing

5   *Negative for methadone on daily script*: Stop script

Reduction or maintenance

Most GPs will have as their long-term aim that the drug user comes off drugs. There is overwhelming evidence that drug users cannot be forced to come off drugs until they are ready to do so, so there is nothing to be gained by imposing a methadone reduction regimen as this is likely to lead to a return to using street drugs. It is important to keep in mind the other important goals of methadone prescribing (see pages 61–2). The evidence suggests that these goals are more likely to be achieved with higher rather than lower doses of methadone and by 'having a treatment goal of successful ongoing maintenance rather than abstinence'.[1]

Prescribing injectables

Recent evidence suggests that 10% of NHS methadone prescriptions are for injectable methadone.[11] The main argument in favour of
prescribing injectables is that some opiate injectors are unwilling or
unable to stop injecting and therefore do not come into oral
methadone programmes. There are however a number of problems
including the risk that injectables be sold and the difficulty in encouraging some users to take oral medication if they know that the doctor
sometimes prescribes injectables. There are undoubtedly a small number of injectors who cannot be helped with oral medication but injectables should only be prescribed by a specialist service or by a GP
with considerable experience in caring for opiate users.

7

Cocaine, amphetamines and designer drugs

Philip Fleming

Introduction

Stimulant users do not often present to GPs for help. Most users take stimulants on a recreational basis. Those who use these drugs heavily and become dependent on them do not see the GP as having anything to offer as a substitute for their illicit drugs. This is in contrast to heroin users, who may present to their GP asking for a methadone script. General practitioners and practice nurses should take the opportunity of broaching the subject of drug use when young people are seen for other health matters.

Approximately one in eight young people between the ages of 16–19 have tried amphetamine and one in ten Ecstasy. Use of these drugs is thus quite common amongst young people. The use of cocaine is less widespread. Only 5% of a sample of 16–25 year olds had tried it. Drug use in general is more common in inner-city areas and particularly on large council estates but it is misleading to try to describe a typical stimulant user as these drugs are often taken as part of a pattern of polydrug misuse.

There are regional variations in stimulant use as reported to the drug misuse databases.[1] Cocaine is most frequently reported in the London area while amphetamine is reported most often in Yorkshire and the South Western regions. Reports from drug workers and the police indicate that amphetamine, cocaine and Ecstasy are readily available from the black market in most areas of England and Wales.

Cocaine

Cocaine is an alkaloid made from the leaves of the coca bush that grows in mountainous regions of South America. It was first isolated in the late nineteenth century and its consumption became widespread in Europe and the USA. Sigmund Freud noted its local anaesthetic and stimulant effects and initially recommended its use as a cure for morphine addiction before realizing its addictive properties.[2]

Cocaine is available in two forms: cocaine hydrochloride and crack cocaine.

Cocaine hydrochloride

Cocaine is produced in the hydrochloride form in illegal laboratories in South America for transport to Europe and the USA. It is an odourless, white, crystalline powder with a bitter taste and is known by various terms including: Charlie, toot, dust and snow. Initially produced with a high purity, by the time it reaches street users it has been mixed with adulterants such as glucose ('cut'), reducing purity to 50%, or less. Cocaine hydrochloride is taken in various ways.

- *Sniffing ('snorting')* – the powder is finely chopped with a razor blade and drawn into two inch-long lines which are then sniffed up one nostril at a time using a straw, or other implement.

- *Injecting* – the hydrochloride is very soluble in water and can easily be prepared for intravenous injection. It is sometimes mixed with heroin and the resultant preparation is called a 'speedball'.

- *Orally* – the most common form is as an elixir in preparations such as the 'Brompton cocktail' used in the treatment of terminally ill patients.

Crack cocaine

Crack cocaine is a purer form of cocaine produced from the hydro-chloride by a simple chemical process involving heating with sodium bicarbonate, usually in the form of baking powder. This separates the alkaloid from the salt and leaves pure, crystalline cocaine that is broken into chunks ('rocks') and sold in small phials or clingfilm 'wraps'. It is known as rock, base or free-base. Crack is usually smoked from 'pipes' (often made from soft drink cans), mixed with tobacco/cannabis, or burnt on a piece of tin foil. It can also be injected but needs to be made soluble first. This is most often done by adding an acid, such as vitamin C.

Epidemiology

There has been an increase in the use of cocaine in Britain over the past ten years, mainly in inner-city areas, with an increase in the use of smokable forms of the drug. However, only a minority of cocaine users present to services. Cocaine notifications were only 2.4% of total notifications in England in 1995,[3] and only 5% of new referrals reported to the regional databases that year were using cocaine as their main drug.[1] 'Snorted' cocaine is used as a recreational drug but is associated with potential development of dependent use. Injected cocaine and smoked crack are very much associated with dependence. Many cocaine users are polydrug users.

Stimulants: cocaine and amphetamine

- *Effects*: elevated mood, increased energy, reduced appetite, raised pulse and blood pressure, dilated pupils

- *Withdrawal symptoms*: depression, craving, irritability, hyperphagia, hypersomnia

- *Adverse effects*: agitation, irritability, restlessness, cardiac arrhythmias, hypertension, convulsions, hallucinations, paranoid psychoses

---

Clinical effects

The acute effects are dose related and the speed of action depends on the route the drug is taken. Thus, taken intravenously or by inhalation the effects develop almost immediately (the 'rush') and if sniffed, within minutes.

Physical effects include a raised pulse rate, blood pressure and temperature and dilatation of the pupils. Tolerance develops to the physical effects of the drug. Very large doses taken by those not used to it can cause hypertension, cardiac arrhythmias and convulsions. Death may occur due to cardiac or respiratory arrest.

Cocaine is a powerful CNS stimulant producing increased energy, wakefulness, activity and an intense feeling of well being. After a single dose these effects taper off after about 30 minutes. Psychological dependence can develop rapidly or over a period of time, with consumption increasing as a result. In some cases a person may use continuously until they are exhausted or run out of the drug (a 'binge' or 'run'), have a drug free period and then binge again.

Increasing use and doses of the drug can result in a number of psychological effects. Visual or tactile hallucinations may occur. Feelings of anxiety and restlessness may lead to suspiciousness and paranoid behaviour. Cocaine psychosis is a toxic state characterized by persecutory delusions and hallucinations occurring in a state of high arousal.

The cocaine abstinence syndrome

The cocaine abstinence syndrome takes different forms.

- The 'crash' is an acute withdrawal state following prolonged or high-dose use in which profound depression and craving occur.

- Withdrawal occurs where there has been regular frequent use and is characterized by fluctuating depression and lack of energy that resolves within days to weeks.

- There may be re-experience of withdrawal symptoms if users are exposed to 'cues' associated with previous usage.

Management

There are not currently any individual treatments that are specifically effective for cocaine use.[4] Few treatment agencies specialize in treating cocaine users, though all should offer help and advice. General advice and information about health risks and safer injecting practices should be given.

Help with withdrawal symptoms may be considered in the more dependent user. Antidepressants can be of help, for example, desipramine 25–50 mg t.d.s. or fluoxetine 20–60 mg mane. Where there is significant agitation, a short-term prescription of diazepam may be given.

Substitute prescribing is not recommended.

Psychological and social support are the mainstays of treatment. More specialized psychological treatments, such as relapse prevention and cue exposure* is available in some centres. Most patients

* The therapist first identifies cues or signals for drug taking, either internal feelings or external events, such as particular places. The drug user is then systematically exposed to these cues and is helped to avoid drug taking in response to them.

can be treated as out-patients, although the most severely dependent may need admission.

Psychiatric complications need to be treated on a symptomatic basis. Paranoid symptoms for example can be treated with neuroleptics, such as haloperidol.

In-patient care will be required for those experiencing extreme distress in acute withdrawal states. Specialist in-patient treatment may be needed for heavy users who are unable to stop taking the drug in the community.

Complementary treatments, such as acupuncture, are being more widely used for cocaine users particularly to help craving and withdrawal. Although there is only limited evidence to support the effectiveness of these treatments in terms of reducing withdrawal symptoms or preventing relapse, when offered they may attract cocaine users into contact with services which they would otherwise avoid.

Amphetamine

This is the general name given to a class of synthetic drugs with adrenaline-like action, known as sympathomimetic amines. Benzedrine, a form of amphetamine sulphate originally sold as a nasal decongestant, was widely used as a stimulant by troops during the Second World War. A number of derivatives of amphetamine such as fenfluramine and phentermine are used as appetite suppressants.

Amphetamine sulphate is the most commonly available substance and is relatively easily made in illegal laboratories in the UK and on the Continent. Known as speed, whizz or sulph, it is an off-white or pinky powder that has always been heavily 'cut' (diluted). The current purity rate is about 5%. It can be swallowed, snorted or dissolved in water and injected.

Recently, a more powerful amphetamine has been appearing on the streets known as 'base' or 'paste'. This is a grey coloured, putty-like substance with a purity of up to 70%, though it is often less than this. It can be taken orally, smoked or injected.

Dexamphetamine sulphate (dexedrine) in tablet form is the only pharmaceutical preparation available.

Methylamphetamine (methedrine) is weight for weight the most potent amphetamine. Known as 'ice' in the USA, it is rarely found in Britain.

Epidemiology

Amphetamine use has been increasing in Britain in recent years; after cannabis it is the most widely used illegal drug. It is used recreationally and particularly as part of the 'dance scene' by young people under the age of 25. Evidence from drug misuse database figures indicates that there are significant numbers of problematic amphetamine users, both those using it as their main drug and polydrug users. About 50% of primary users presenting to services inject the drug.[1]

Clinical effects

Amphetamine is a powerful CNS stimulant producing an elevated mood and making the user feel energetic, alert and self-confident. Feelings of hunger and fatigue are reduced and there is increased talkativeness, restlessness and sometimes agitation. Some individuals become anxious and irritable.

As a sympathomimetic drug it causes increased heart rate and blood pressure, palpitations, dilated pupils, dry mouth and sweating. Acute intoxication is characterized by dizziness, sweating, chest pain, palpitations and cardiac arrhythmias. Body temperature may be raised and convulsions may occur.

Tolerance develops to the mood-elevating effects of the drug and also to many of the physical effects. It is not uncommon for heavy users to take several grams a day. Some users may take the drug on a repeated basis for two or three days ('speed run') ending when the supply or user is 'spent'.

A number of adverse psychological effects may result from amphetamine use and these are in general dose related. Individuals may become increasingly paranoid, believing they are being watched or followed. They can experience vivid visual or auditory hallucinations. A full-blown paranoid psychosis may develop (the amphetamine psychosis), which may be indistinguishable from schizophrenia. Another complication of chronic amphetamine use is automatic stereotyped behaviour: for example, repeatedly taking apart and putting together a radio. These symptoms usually remit within a few days of stopping the drug.

Withdrawal symptoms do occur particularly after regular or high dose use. Abrupt withdrawal after a binge is followed by fatigue, depression, hunger and a need to sleep. Cessation after long-term use is often accompanied by feelings of lassitude and mild depression that may take some weeks to resolve.

Management of cocaine and amphetamine use

- No specific treatments are available

- Psychological and social support are the mainstays of management

- Advice and information should be given about the health risks and safer injecting practices

- Use of antidepressants for withdrawal symptoms

- Symptomatic treatment for psychiatric complications

- Psychological methods: relapse prevention and cue exposure

- Complementary therapies may encourage users into treatment

Management

There is no specific treatment for amphetamine misuse. General advice and information should be given about health risks. For those injecting the drug, advice about safer injecting practices and where to obtain clean needles and syringes should be given.

Those heavy or long-term users who experience withdrawal symptoms can be helped with an antidepressant, such as desipramine 25–50 mg t.d.s. or fluoxetine 20–60 mg mane, which may need to be continued for several weeks.

Patients who are agitated and restless, or who are showing psychotic symptoms, will need treatment with neuroleptics such as haloperidol. Admission to a psychiatric unit may be required if symptoms are persistent and severe.

Amphetamine prescribing

- Controversial treatment

- No scientific evidence of efficacy

- Should only be undertaken with specialist support

- Only consider for heavy dependent users as a harm-reduction measure

---

Substitution treatment

Substitution treatment for amphetamine use is a controversial issue since scientific evidence for its efficacy does not exist as it does for methadone treatment. It is advised that any prescription of amphetamine should be undertaken together with the local specialist drug service. It should only be considered for heavy, dependent users, particularly injecting users, as a harm-reduction measure.[5] There should be clear evidence of amphetamine use by urine testing and at least a six-month history of daily use. It is contraindicated if there is any history of mental illness, hypertension, heart disease or if the patient is pregnant. Dexamphetamine sulphate (Dexedrine) can be prescribed as 5 mg tablets, or the pharmacist can make up a suspension. The aim is not to give an equivalent dose to that used illegally but to minimize withdrawal symptoms and craving and it is recommended that a maximum of 60 mg a day is prescribed to be taken in the morning. Prescriptions should be given at no longer than weekly intervals and preferably daily, or two or three times a week. Patients should be regularly monitored for use of other drugs, injecting behaviour, mental state and general social stability. If there is no improvement in any of these measures the treatment should be ceased. Long-term maintenance prescribing of amphetamine is not recommended. The aim should be to stabilize the drug user over six to nine months and then reduce and stop the prescription.

Designer drugs

The term designer drugs originally referred to illicit substances that were pharmacologically similar to drugs of abuse controlled by national and international legislation but they differed in chemical structure so that they remained out of reach of the law.

Ecstasy

- Widely used recreational drug

- Stimulant and hallucinogenic effects

- Physical effects include: dry mouth, tachycardia, dilated pupils, facial muscle stiffness

- Adverse psychological effects include: anxiety, depression, panic, flashbacks, psychotic states

- Deaths have been reported after using Ecstasy

Ecstasy

This is one of a group of analogues of MDA (methylenedioxy-amphetamine), the so-called hallucinogenic amphetamines; of which the best known is 3,4-methylenedioxymethylamphetamine (MDMA), known as Ecstasy.

First developed in 1914 as an appetite suppressant, Ecstasy was used as an adjunct to psychotherapy in the US in the 1970s before being used as a recreational drug in the 1980s. It first appeared in the UK in 1985 and its use spread widely in the early 1990s.

Known as 'E' and many other names depending on the colour and shape, it is supplied as a pill or capsule, which is swallowed. Typically, a single tablet is taken, but some users may take several during the course of an evening and there are some reports of as many as ten tablets being taken in an evening. Analysis of tablets seized by the police shows they are often contaminated with MDMA analogues or substances such as lysergic acid diethylamide (LSD), ketamine or amphetamine.

Epidemiology

Ecstasy is relatively widely used on a recreational basis by young people as one of the 'dance' drugs.[6] It came to prominence because of its use in 'rave' parties and now it is more widely used in clubs and private parties. It is most commonly used at weekends.

Clinical effects

The drug has stimulant and hallucinogenic effects. There is a general enhancement of sensory perceptions, visual illusions and states of altered consciousness. Users describe a feeling of empathy and non-sexual affection towards others. The stimulant effects, which seem to be more prominent with higher doses, are similar to those of amphetamine. The effects of a single dose can last for up to four hours.

Common physical effects include tachycardia, dry mouth, dilated pupils, facial muscle stiffness and parasthesiae.

A number of deaths have been reported in recreational users – the figure for 1994 was ten. This figure should be taken in the context of the estimated three million doses of the drug that are taken annually. By comparison, some 28 000 deaths annually are attributed to alcohol. Deaths caused by Ecstasy are not related to the dose of drug taken. A form of disseminated intravascular coagulation may occur as a result of heatstroke caused by a direct effect on thermoregulation and vigorous dancing in high ambient temperatures. A few users have died of the stimulant effects on the heart or from cerebrovascular accidents because of raised blood pressure. There are also recorded deaths from water intoxication when users have drunk water excessively to counter imagined dehydration.

Several adverse psychological effects have been described: these include anxiety states, depression, panic disorder, flashbacks and psychotic episodes.[7] These adverse effects tend to occur more often in heavy users. There is some debate as to whether the use of Ecstasy can lead to damage to 5-HT neurones in the brain and that this may be responsible for adverse psychological effects.

Advice to Ecstasy users

- Take only one tablet an evening

- Do not mix with other drugs or alcohol

- If dancing, take regular breaks to cool down and drink a pint of fluid each hour

Management

There are no specific treatments for Ecstasy use. Advice and information about the drug and possible adverse effects should be given. If young people are going to take the drug they should limit the amount taken (preferably to only one tablet), not mix it with other drugs or alcohol, take breaks from dancing to cool down and drink a pint of fluid each hour. They should understand the need to drink fluids to counteract dehydration, not the effects of the drug.

Adverse psychological effects should be treated symptomatically. Users should be advised to avoid the use of all psychoactive substances for several weeks. Persistent depressive symptoms probably respond best to selective serotonin re-uptake inhibitors (SSRIs), such as fluoxetine.

Leaflets about drugs misuse aimed at parents and young people may be obtained free of charge from the Health Education Authority, Drugs Campaign Ordering Service, PO Box 105, Sandwich, Kent, CT13 9BR. Tel: 01304 614 737; Fax: 01304 617 727.

Acknowledgement

Thanks are due to Andrew Preston for his helpful comments.

8

Use and abuse of benzodiazepines by polydrug users

Chris Ford

Introduction

Benzodiazepines were first introduced into clinical practice in the 1960s. Diazepam was amongst the first in 1963, followed by nitrazepam (1965), temazepam (1977) and flunitrazepam in 1982. They soon became the drug treatment of choice in anxiety and insomnia, favoured over barbiturates because they were thought to be reliable, have less side-effects, be less addictive and appeared safer in overdose.

By the 1970s, they were being favourably received by patients and doctors and became widely prescribed. In some countries they were available without prescription and were used even more extensively. They had enormous commercial profitability that led to the development of almost a hundred different brands, 20 of which gained common usage in the UK. The high point of use in the UK was about 1980 with use decreasing since.

More recently, it has become clear that benzodiazepine use by illicit drug users, particularly opiate users, is a major problem in and out of treatment. This problem has been to an extent overshadowed by the concerns raised by their prescribed use in women and the elderly. As use in these groups decreases, it is likely that illicit drug users will become the largest groups of users of benzodiazepines.[1] This is a major clinical and public health problem that needs to be addressed.

Benzodiazepine dependency

The first warnings that benzodiazepine use can result in dependency date back to 1963. The medical profession took little notice of these

reports and decided that because benzodiazepines were safe in overdose, they could not really cause many problems. There was also
enormous commercial pressure to prescribe these drugs which were
regarded as a universal panacea to patients' anxieties. Consequently
the extent and nature of dependency was not defined until several
years after the initial warnings.[2] Eventually the problems of dependence were recognized and there is now a wealth of literature on the
use and abuse of benzodiazepines, normal dose dependency and withdrawal symptoms.

The Safety of Medicines Committee produced a systematic review
of benzodiazepines in 1980.[3] The Royal College of Psychiatrists stated
that they should only be used when insomnia and/or anxiety was
severe, disabling and causing extreme distress.[4]

Benzodiazepines can produce two types of dependence.

1   *Therapeutic dependence* – mitigates suffering in long-term anxiety,
    which may be acceptable to GP and patient (the poor analogy to
    the use of insulin in the diabetic patient has been used).

2   *Morbid dependency* – escalating dosage, in order to avoid with-
    drawal symptoms.

It has also been found that dependency, as evidenced by withdrawal
symptoms when the patient attempts to stop the drug, can occur at
normal doses. There are large differences in benzodiazepine potency,
and the half-lives of these drugs vary from two hours to 100 hours.
Triazolam and lorazepam are two benzodiazepines that cause high
dependency.

Control of prescribing

All benzodiazepines were classified as prescription-only medicines
under the Medicines Act 1968. They can only be prescribed by
doctors and dispensed from a pharmacy. Under the Misuse of Drugs
Act 1971 they are defined as a class C drug. Since 1986, under this
Act, unauthorized supply is an offence, as is the illicit production of
these drugs.

Temazepam was reclassified as a controlled drug in 1996 to help
prevent extensive use by illicit drug users.

Therapeutic use of benzodiazepines

Advantages

- Highly effective in the short term

- Rapid onset of action

- Toxicity is low – few side-effects when in use

- Safe in overdose

Disadvantages

- Underlying cause of anxiety is not addressed. Supportive counselling has been shown to work equally well[5]

- Tolerance to the drug can develop after only a few days

- 'Rebound insomnia' – on ceasing the drug, sleep can become more difficult than before

- Dependency can develop quickly and easily

- Withdrawal symptoms can occur

- Hangover effects in the morning when used for sleep

- Psychomotor impairment may develop rapidly

- Major and minor somatic illnesses are increased

- If prescribed and not used by the patient, diversion to the illicit market is a possibility

Although the disadvantages of prescribing benzodiazepines are well known there are still over 14 million prescriptions of benzodiazepines issued annually worldwide.

Illicit use of benzodiazepines

Non-medical use of benzodiazepines has become an increasing problem. An example of their use has been seen in Glasgow, where the injecting of temazepam capsules ('jellies') resulted in a marked increase in mortality and morbidity in young people. In 1989, this eventually led the manufacturers of temazepam capsules to change the contents from a liquid to those filled with wax. It was soon discovered that the wax could be cooked and the resultant liquid injected. This led to a range of medical problems from blocked blood vessels sometimes resulting in limb amputation due to gangrene. All capsules were withdrawn in 1996 and now only tablets can be prescribed, although capsules can still be bought on the street.

In the UK in 1993, benzodiazepine use (excluding those in whom a benzodiazepine was their first drug of choice) was reported by 16% of illicit drug users. Their use was highest in dihydrocodeine users (28.5%) and methadone users (23.8%), less common in amphetamine users (13.6%) and heroin users (11.4%).[6] Different studies from around the world have shown different rates of benzodiazepine use by illicit drug users, ranging from between 32% and 73% in injecting drug users.

The use of benzodiazepines by young people is also increasing. In a 1995 report, 41% of 15 year olds had been offered them and 5% had tried them.[7]

Illicit drug users use benzodiazepines for their tranquillizing and hypnotic effects and to reduce anxiety. Anxiety may arise from underlying psychological problems or the effects of other drugs being used, such as stimulants. Insomnia can be a real problem and may be worse when trying to stabilize or reduce other illicit drug use. Benzodiazepines are also taken to suppress depression and reduce 'voices' in the head, which may result from the use of drugs such as stimulants and cocaine. They are also used to cushion the depressant effects of cocaine, which occur after the intense, but short-lived high.

Benzodiazepines are taken orally or intravenously. Temazepam particularly is injected.[8] Users can get a 'rush' or 'high' on benzodiazepines and this is greater when they are injected. These users are usually taking other illicit drugs, most commonly opiates. They tend to be younger and use much higher doses, sometimes up to 50 times the therapeutic doses, with five or ten times the normal dose being commonplace.[9] Polydrug users taking methadone or other opiates usually take their benzodiazepines at the same time, to increase the 'rush' or pleasurable effect.

Research also appears to demonstrate that opiate users who also use benzodiazepines are more psychologically and socially impaired than other opiate users and have higher rates of crime involvement. They have also been found to be more difficult to treat.[1] Insufficient attention to benzodiazepine dependency and/or withdrawal may result in poor outcomes if opiate users are attempting to detoxify from opiates.

There is higher HIV risk-taking behaviour amongst people who are also taking benzodiazepines. This includes increased sharing of equipment, with an increased number of people.[1] There is higher incidence of hepatitis C infection, which itself is an indicator of increased sharing. Benzodiazepine users are also shown to have injected more frequently and to use a greater mixture of drugs. Casual sexual contacts and episodes of unprotected sexual intercourse are also increased.

Illicit benzodiazepine use

Positive effects for the user

- Cheap, legal, available
- Function better, cope with life, calmer, sleep better
- Treat heroin withdrawal/comedown from stimulant
- 'Putting the rod back' into methadone for intoxication
- Enhances the effects of other drugs

Associated harms

- Unsafe injecting
- Tolerance
- Withdrawal fits
- Role in overdose in association with alcohol/opiates
- Increased craving for other drugs
- Obtained on prescription – doctor shopping
- Memory problems
- Paradoxical aggression
- Child-protection issues
- Poor social functioning, 'zombies'
- Need to finance the habit leads to crime
- Economic problems

Users can show extreme behaviour changes with aggression, increased hostility and antisocial acts when they binge on benzodiazepines, or their supply is interrupted. Withdrawal fits can occur when withdrawing or ceasing high doses.

Withdrawal symptoms

Withdrawal symptoms when trying to decrease use of benzodiazepines are multiple and varied. The symptoms are similar, but more severe, in high dose. Unfortunately no drugs have been found to help alleviate withdrawal symptoms.[10]

Patients and doctors may interpret some of these symptoms as a return to the pre-existing anxiety state. The symptoms of withdrawal usually last over a period of weeks, but a substantial minority of users have a protracted withdrawal course[11] and one third of patients report significant symptoms ten months to three-and-a-half years following withdrawal.[12]

Withdrawal symptoms experienced by patients vary according to the type of benzodiazepine being used. Longer-acting benzodiazepines, such as diazepam, are less difficult to withdraw from than short-acting preparations, such as lorazepam. If withdrawal is abrupt, between 58–100% of users have some degree of withdrawal syndrome, which is worse if high doses have been taken.[9] If withdrawal is gradual, there is still a high reportage of withdrawal symptoms, but

---

Benzodiazepine withdrawal symptoms

Psychological symptoms

- Drowsiness, fatigue, poor memory

- Excitability, unreality, depersonalization

- Perceptual distortion, hallucinations

- Craving for the drug

- Phobias, anxiety, panic attacks

- Depression

- Paranoid thoughts, rage, aggression

Benzodiazepine withdrawal symptoms

Somatic symptoms

1 *Central nervous system*
- Headache, all over pain
- 'Pins and needles', 'crawling in the skin'
- Weakness, tremor, ataxia
- Muscle twitches, fasciculation
- Dizziness, light-headedness
- Blurred, or double, vision
- Tinnitus, speech difficulty
- Hypersensitive to noise, light, smell, touch, taste
- Insomnia, nightmares, fits

2 *Gastrointestinal*
- Nausea, vomiting, abdominal pain
- Diarrhoea or constipation
- Appetite or weight change
- Dry mouth, metallic taste

3 *Cardiovascular or respiratory*
- Flushing, sweating
- Palpitations, racing pulse

4 *Urogenital or endocrine*
- Thirst, frequency, polyuria
- Incontinence, menorrhagia
- Mammary pain or swelling

5 *Miscellaneous*
- Rash, itching
- Stuffy nose, sinusitis
- Influenza-like symptoms

these are less severe than with abrupt withdrawal. The number of people experiencing withdrawal symptoms is higher in the second half of the tapering dose.

Factors affecting the withdrawal reaction

- Duration of benzodiazepine use – if taken for eight or more months the withdrawal syndrome is eight times more likely. If the use has been over three years there is a reaction in 50% of users, and in 75% if the use has been for longer than six years

- Increased reaction if user has a history of other drug use and/or alcohol use and/or social problems

- Speed of withdrawal from the drug

- New symptoms and the re-emergence of symptoms can arise during withdrawal

- Withdrawal symptoms are greater if attempting to come off several drugs at once

---

Substitute prescribing

Whether GPs should institute substitute prescribing of benzodiazepines is still a debated issue. Substitute prescribing can be seen as a harm-reduction strategy. It is argued that it may help patients stabilize their lifestyle and drug use, and removes them from the illicit market. It acknowledges that these drugs are a large problem for many polydrug users and offering a script can attract them into services. There is physical dependence on benzodiazepines for which there is a suitable long-acting preparation to prescribe as a substitute that can relieve withdrawal problems. However there are other considerations to be taken into account, and the advisability of substitute prescribing for a patient depends upon a careful assessment of the likely benefits weighed against the possible disadvantages. Some GPs feel more comfortable prescribing a benzodiazepine than methadone, because it is a drug with which they feel familiar and it is not a controlled drug. In general, GPs should be more *unwilling* to initiate a benzodiazepine script than opiate prescribing because of the possible attendant problems.

Substitute benzodiazepine prescribing should only be considered if the following conditions are met.

1 There is evidence of dependency from the history and symptoms.

2 The goals of any substitute prescribing have been established, or are being worked toward. They include:

    – stabilization of patient's lifestyle

    – stabilization of drug use

    – patients' ability to remove themselves from the illicit drug market.

3 The drug user is taking benzodiazepines daily.

4 Urine screens confirm the presence of benzodiazepines. (The drugs may be detected in the urine up to three to four weeks after ingestion.)

5 Concurrent opiate misuse has been stabilized with prescribed methadone.

Issues in substitute prescribing

- There is a high risk of dependency

- Coming off benzodiazepines is more difficult than coming off opiates

- Very high risk of withdrawal symptoms that increase with duration of use

- Extensive tissue damage and risk of death can occur if tablets are injected

- Can be used in exchange for other drugs on the street

- Side-effects and long-term problems may not be understood by the user

Reducing-dose prescribing

This is the preferred option if a decision to prescribe has been agreed with the patient. The following procedure should be adopted.

1   Only prescribe one benzodiazepine at a time.

2   If the patient is using more than one benzodiazepine, change to one preparation.

3   Change all benzodiazepines being used to diazepam, because of its stability and longer half-life. Prescribing of benzodiazepines other than diazepam is very rarely appropriate.

4   Keep other drugs, such as methadone, stable while reducing benzodiazepines.

5   Monitor patient carefully for concurrent psychiatric problems that may come to light as the dose is reduced.

How to change from one benzodiazepine to another

- Convert all other benzodiazepines to the equivalent dose of diazepam to minimize withdrawal symptoms

- Make all the change at the same time, unless the patient is very anxious, when it should be made over three to four weeks

Benzodiazepine equivalents

Diazepam (Valium) 10 mg is equivalent to:

- temazepam, 20 mg (Euhypnos, 'jellies')

- nitrazepam, 10 mg (Mogadon, 'moggies')

- lorazepam, 1 mg (Ativan)

- oxazepam, 30 mg (Serenid-D)

- chlordiazepoxide, 20 mg (Librium)

- flurazepam, 30 mg (Dalmane)

- flunitrazepam, 1 mg (Rohypnol) (Not on NHS drugs list)

Calculating required dose of diazepam

1 Starting

- Aim at the lowest dose that is possible.
- Start at 20–30 mg daily of diazepam.
- There is rarely a need to start above 40 mg diazepam daily.

2 Divide up the daily dose

- Keep some of the dose for helping sleep at night.
- The patient should not be 'stoned' or drowsy during the day.

3 Review after one week

- If withdrawals are occurring, increase the dose in steps of 5–10 mg, every one to two weeks.
- Doses above 60 mg are rarely needed.

Reducing the diazepam dose

1 If drug users are taking more than 30 mg of diazepam, start reducing by 5 mg per month.

2 If drug users are using very large doses (above 60 mg), the first half of the dose can be withdrawn more quickly.

3 Users may need to be in-patients if they have been taking large doses, especially during pregnancy.

4 Reduction of the dose can be quicker if there has been a short history of use.

5 When 20 mg is reached, or if the drug user has only been taking 20 mg or less, the withdrawal regimen can be 1 mg every one to two weeks.

6 When a dose of 5 mg is reached, a reduction of 0.5 mg every two weeks is usually effective in minimizing withdrawal symptoms.

7 The reduction should not be fixed but titrated against the patient's withdrawal symptoms.

8   Reduction may need to be slower if the user is experiencing withdrawal.

9   While reducing, counselling, support groups and relaxation techniques can be helpful.

It is important to note that because of long-term effects, patients on a benzodiazepine script must be regularly reviewed.

Dispensing by the pharmacist

This should be done daily when prescribing is first started. The blue daily dispensing form, MDA FP10 (England and Wales), cannot be used because benzodiazepines are not class A notifiable drugs, but prescriptions can be generated on a daily basis on the practice computer. The patient should be encouraged to use the same named pharmacist for all dispensing. The GP should discuss the scripting policy with the pharmacist who may be willing to dispense daily on an FP10 prescription. Lost prescriptions should not be replaced, and neither should a shortfall in tablets because of the risks of over use before the next routine appointment.

Other drugs to help in reduction

If insomnia continues to be a problem, the use of a non-benzodiazepine hypnotic for a short period (two weeks) can be helpful, e.g. chloral betaine 707 mg 1–2 nocte, thioridazine 25–50 mg nocte or promethazine 25–50 mg nocte.

Antidepressants may also be helpful for sleep and can be used longer term, e.g. amitryptyline 25–75 mg nocte or dothiepin 75–100 mg nocte, although abuse of diothiepin has been reported.

Maintenance prescribing

Maintenance prescribing of benzodiazepines is controversial and has not been shown to have any definite 'medical' value, unlike methadone maintenance which has been shown to reduce injecting and risk behaviour in illicit drug users. However, the arguments put forward in support of reduction prescribing of benzodiazepines may also be used to justify maintenance prescribing in users who are unable to accept, or manage, with a reducing script (see Table 8.1). These arguments are similar to those for maintenance prescribing of methadone, and possibly amphetamines.

Benefits of maintenance prescribing

- Acknowledges that these drugs are a significant problem to many polydrug users.

- May achieve the goals of long-term prescribing.

- Can be seen as a harm-reduction strategy, as it is for opiates.

- Helps to reduce relapse into illicit use and removes drug users from the illicit market.

- HIV and other infections are more common in opiate users also using illicit benzodiazepines.

- Relieves withdrawal problems.

- Less stigma – prescribing of benzodiazepines may be seen as more socially acceptable.

Table 8.1: Rationale for longer term prescribing of substitute drugs[9]

	Benzodiazepines	Opiates	Amphetamine
Social reasons – stabilize lifestyle, less crime, etc.	+	+	+
Attract into medical services	+	+	+
Substitute used produces safe effect	+	+	x
Physical dependence on drug of misuse	+	+	?
Long-acting substitute available to prescribe, enhancing stability	+	+	x

Disadvantages of maintenance prescribing

- Problems of dependence, tolerance and abuse.

- Withdrawal symptoms worsen with longer use.

- Doctors may prescribe benzodiazepines more readily than metha-done. This may be inappropriate if opiate use is not also stabilized.

- Risk of diversion of prescribed drugs into the illicit market.

- Overdose can be dangerous, especially in conjunction with other drugs.

- Risk of injection of tablets.

If maintenance prescribing is undertaken, the smallest dose possible of diazepam should be administered. Maintenance prescribing should be seen as a last option and should be integrated into a treat-ment plan with goals drawn up in conjunction with the patient.

Summary

The use of benzodiazepines by polydrug users is a growing clinical and public health problem that needs to be addressed. Whether benzodiazepines should be prescribed at all, on a reduction pro-gramme or as a maintenance dose, is still a matter for debate.

There are no data on the efficacy of long-term benzodiazepine prescribing comparable to that for methadone maintenance. We also know that benzodiazepine use is associated with greater risk-taking, although the relationship is still unclear.

A suitable plan of treatment for polydrug users in general prac-tice is first to establish a user on the right amount of methadone. If there are continuing problems with illicit use of benzodiazepines, try an increased methadone dose before considering benzodiazepine prescribing.

If the drug user has a confirmed problem with benzodiazepines spend the necessary time explaining the problems of these drugs, their withdrawal symptoms and the risks of on-going use.

When this has been done, convert to one benzodiazepine, and draw up a reduction programme as described earlier in the text. Titrate the dose reduction against the patient and aim for eventual abstinence from benzodiazepines. Leave the methadone at an agreed dose while this is being undertaken.

If reduction is not accepted or managed, then maintenance on one long-acting benzodiazepine, at the smallest dose possible, can be considered. This is a last option and should be fitted into a treatment plan with goals drawn up in conjunction with the patient.

9

Safer injection, safer use, safer sex: a harm-minimization approach

Clare Gerada, James Tighe and Clive Barrett

Introduction

General practitioners are ideally placed to reduce the potential harm that illicit drug use can cause to an individual. The surgery is often the first port of call for the drug user and his or her family seeking advice. Even if the primary health care team is reluctant to offer sub-stitute prescribing, general medical services including advice about safer drug use should be available to all attending for help. Whilst illicit drug use can never be safe it can be made safer. Advising users to use more safely is not sanctioning drug use, only limiting the harm caused by that use. This chapter focuses on help the primary health care team can give to reduce the morbidity and mortality caused by illicit drug use and related behaviours.

Safer injecting

Complications associated with drug use can occur either directly from the drug itself, such as overdose, or indirectly from dangers associated with the route of use, in particular injecting use.

Drug-related complications

Drugs obtained on the street are rarely pure and are frequently 'cut' with other substances, some innocuous, such as talcum powder, others more dangerous, such as vim or quinine. The injecting route has the least margin of error if the purity of the street drug is inadvertently high.

Injecting drug use complications

Technique-specific

- Abscesses

- Cellulitis

- Embolic events/deep vein thrombosis

Sharing

- HIV/AIDS

- Hepatitis

General

- Anaemia

- Poor nutrition

- Menstrual irregularities

- Dental caries

Overdose of sedative drugs leads to respiratory depression: hypo-thermia and coma can result. Basic advice about knowing your dealer, not using alone, reducing 'normal' dose after a period of abstinence, the correct recovery position if a friend is found uncon-scious and immediate summoning of an ambulance can save lives. Equipping injecting opiate users with preloaded syringes of naloxone may be the greatest harm reduction intervention a GP can make. This intervention is not currently in practice but is worth debate despite obvious controversies.[1]

Heroin is the drug most often associated with injecting use, although almost all other commonly abused drugs can be injected either in a form designed for parenteral use or by crushing tables or by direct injection of the oral liquid formulation. If the substance injected has not fully dissolved or if the liquid is viscous, such as that contained in temazepam gel-filled capsules ('jellies'), embolic events can occur leading to thrombosis and gangrene.

The prescribing GP must always be aware of the potential harm any prescribed drug can cause, especially if injected. Drug users should be prescribed liquid rather than tablet formulations of 'at risk' substances, such as analgesics and benzodiazepines.

Route-specific complications

Injecting drug use carries the greatest risk of infection. Injecting equipment is frequently shared or cursorily cleaned. Dirty and unhygienic injecting habits can result in local or systemic infections and poor injecting technique can cause venous or arterial thrombosis. The harm associated with injecting drug use can be reduced by correcting poor injecting technique, providing clean needles and syringes via needle or pharmacy exchange schemes and by giving correct advice on cleaning injecting equipment.

Safer injecting use

- Always inject with blood flow

- Rotate injecting sites

- Use smallest bore needle possible

- Avoid neck, breast, feet and hand veins

- Mix powders with sterile water and filter solution before injecting

- Always dispose of equipment safely (either in a bin provided or by placing the needle inside the syringe and placing both inside a drinks can)

- Avoid injecting into infected areas

- Do not inject into swollen limbs, even if the veins appear to be distended

- Poor veins means poor technique. Try to see what is going wrong

- Do not use alone

Some of the most common harmful practices arise from ignorance, such as injecting towards rather than away from the hand when using the outside of the forearm (therefore against the flow of blood) or using contaminated paraphernalia (spoon, filter) believing only clean needles and syringes are needed to avoid infections.

Cleaning injecting equipment

The following are needed to bleach clean injecting equipment:

- needle and syringe
- thin, undiluted household bleach
- clean, cold water
- two clean cups, or wide-topped bottles

Method

1   Pour bleach into one cup (or bottle) and water into another

2   Draw bleach up with the dirty needle and syringe

3   Expel bleach into toilet or sink

4   Repeat steps 2 and 3

5   Draw water up through needle and syringe

6   Expel water into toilet or sink

7   Repeat steps 5 and 6 at least once, ideally twice or three times

Points to remember when cleaning equipment

- Boiling plastic syringes melts them
- Thick bleach is impossible to draw up through a needle
- Cold water is recommended as warm water may encourage blood to coagulate and hence will be harder to expel through the needle

---

Injecting drug users and their partners should be offered hepatitis B testing and immunization, and hepatitis C testing.

Safer drug use

Snorting, smoking or swallowing drugs, though safer than injecting, are not administration routes entirely without risk. The simplicity of enteral (swallowing, drinking) drug use increases the possibility of experimentation, either through mixing drugs or taking large quantities.

Dangerous drug interactions can occur between drugs that affect the central nervous system such as alcohol, opiates and benzodiazepines. The young and naïve user in search of the elusive 'high' may be tempted to consume drug cocktails, each drug not expected to produce psychogenic effects separately. This is particularly the case for methadone, which taken alone or in combination with other drugs can end in death from overdose. All new prescriptions for methadone must be accompanied with a warning about the danger of overdose and of mixing with alcohol or benzodiazepines. Prescribing methadone on a daily dispensing basis, and limiting doses to no more than 40 mg per day until the user's tolerance is known are important interventions the GP can make to reduce the potential harm of the drug. If unsure about prescribing, do not prescribe; opiate withdrawal does not cause death.

Safer drug use – advice to the non-injector

- Know what you are taking
- Using cocktails of drugs can be more dangerous than single drug use
- Use a safer route; snorting, smoking or swallowing are usually safer than injecting
- Look after yourself; eating, sleeping, exercise, rest

Inhaling drugs is less hazardous than any other route but still is not completely safe. Hot smoke, if not cooled first, can burn the bronchial tissues, and inhaled heroin or cocaine can precipitate and worsen asthma. Purified cocaine is usually smoked in a glass water pipe and

produces a sudden intense 'high' comparable to that produced by
intravenous use. The effects subside very rapidly and leave the user
craving for another dose. Inhalations may be repeated as often as
every few minutes and can continue for many hours. Overdose of
cocaine can result from inhaled use, the physical effects being hypertension and hyperthermia. High dosage or repeated use can lead to
death.

Substances such as solvents and amyl-nitrite do not need to be
heated to have their psychoactive effects; indeed their flammability
makes applying a flame very dangerous. When inhaling volatile substances it is important that there is an adequate supply of air reaching
the lungs together with the vapour. Again, users should be advised
not to use alone and to use in safe places, i.e. not roof-tops or near
river banks.

Snorting of drugs is the most uncommon route of use and is normally associated with powdered cocaine and amphetamine. Prolonged
use in this way can cause atrophy of the nasal septum and resulting
breathing difficulties.

What advice can be given to someone taking a substance of unknown nature and dosage? For some users this uncertainty is part of
the 'buzz' of using illicit drugs, though most would like to know what
and how much of a drug they are taking. For Ecstasy users, some drug
outreach services provide education clinics at rave parties that can
include sample testing of tablets to confirm they are Ecstasy. General
practitioners may need to acknowledge a young person's experimental drug use, pointing out the risks of taking unknown drugs at parties,
of mixing drugs and alcohol and the dangers of 'spiking' drinks.
Advice about the need to keep cool and maintaining an adequate
fluid intake at parties should also be stressed.

The psychotropic effects of some drugs, especially hallucinogenic
drugs, such as cannabis and LSD, are partly dependent on the expectations and pre-existing mood of the user, and so may exacerbate
pre-existing anxiety or depression. It is not advisable therefore to use
these drugs when alone.

Safer sex

The issue of safer sex is much more difficult for GPs or nurses to
discuss with their patients. Many professionals feel uncomfortable in
talking about sexual issues, especially when it comes to discussing

homosexual and non-penetrative sexual practices. Whilst most GPs may not be able to discuss in detail the relative risks of the various types of sexual activity, they should be able to offer some advice and where appropriate direct a patient to another source of information, e.g. Terrence Higgins Trust, local genito-urinary medicine clinic.

Whilst injecting drug users and their consorts are undoubtedly at risk of sexually transmitted diseases, such as HIV infection or hepatitis, they are by no means the only at-risk group. In order to overcome clumsiness in bringing up the issue of safer sex with patients it should become common practice to discuss the issue with all patients presenting, for example, for family planning checks or travel immunizations. The new patient registration check includes taking a cervical smear history, an ideal opportunity to discuss current sexual practice with women. With men, this can also be included, as a routine, when discussing other health promotion issues, such as alcohol and smoking consumption. Where condoms are given, time should be taken to explain the correct use. This should be a practical demonstration using fingers or a plastic model.

Safer sex guide

- Limit number of sexual partners

- Ideally, be monogamous with current partner

- Avoid anal intercourse, oral/anal contact and insertion of objects or hand into anus

- Use condoms for penetrative sex

- If condom use not possible, a diaphragm, which offers some protection, should be considered

- Remember hepatitis infection can be transmitted through body fluids, such as saliva

---

Summary

The primary care team must be prepared to match the expectations and needs of the patient at time of presentation, agree on realistic goals and gently facilitate change in behaviour in the direction of safer drug use. Setting unrealistic conditions before helping drug users, for example, insisting that they are drug-free before providing hepatitis B vaccination, will only result in failure, demoralizing GP and patient alike. Working on other aspects of harm reduction and highlighting success in areas such as not sharing needles/syringes or not injecting into thrombosed veins may restore self-esteem and bring about unexpected benefits in other areas.

10

Caring for the pregnant drug user

Chris Ford and Mary Hepburn

Introduction

Patterns of drug use by men and women are changing. The number of women using drugs has risen over the past few years, with almost a 500% increase in notifications in the last two decades.[1] Eighty per cent of women users presenting to agencies in 1995 were aged between 15 and 34, representing a sizeable number in their childbearing years.[2]

No good data exist on the incidence of drug use by pregnant women. Studies of antenatal urine screening for drugs give figures of 3–5% of women showing positive for illicit drugs, mainly amphetamines, cannabinoids and opiates.[3]

Much of the data about numbers of women drug users are incomplete and overlapping, but as well as an increase in notifications, there seems to be an increase in women who use drugs in custody, acute medical admissions of women using drugs and deaths. Women tend to hide their drug use more. This may be because women who use drugs tend to get more social disapproval than men. Society often views women drug users as deviant, unfit, lonely and isolated from their families. This stereotype of a women drug user is rarely true.

Women in general attend their GP more than men and are usually familiar with this environment. Women drug users may prefer seeing their GP for their drug problems as well as other health problems. GPs may know them long before they become pregnant.

Drug use and fertility

The use of illicit drugs on a regular basis can theoretically affect fertility in a number of ways. It may cause weight loss and amenorrhoea with anovulation. An increased incidence of pelvic inflammatory disease in drug users, particularly those supporting their habit by prostitution is probably also significant. However, amenorrhoea cannot be regarded as an indication of inability to conceive, and effective contraception is still essential. Women using drugs may plan to conceive, or become pregnant by accident. Starting treatment with substitute opiates, such as methadone, is a time when fertility increases so offering contraception and/or preconception counselling needs to go hand in hand with the beginning of treatment for the drug problem.

Preconception counselling

If women drug users are being seen in general practice, the GP has an excellent opportunity to provide preconception counselling. This needs to include – discussion of good nutrition, folic acid use to prevent neural tube defects, discussion of the risks of smoking and alcohol, rubella immunity check, ascertainment of hepatitis B status and taking a cervical smear if needed.

In addition the effects of illicit drugs in pregnancy, on the woman and the fetus, can be discussed. Information should be given to allow the woman to make decisions from a position of knowledge. She can then be helped with her decisions, even if they are different from the ones others would have made. Testing for HIV and hepatitis C infection can be offered, if the woman is counselled appropriately. Pregnancy can put an additional strain on a drug user. Some women stop using, others become more chaotic or increase their drug use during this time. Achieving stability or abstinence prior to pregnancy is time well spent.

Pregnant women who use drugs

All pregnant women, whether they use drugs or not, have mixed feelings about a forthcoming child – will it be normal? Will he or she love me? Am I/can I be a good mother? It should be remembered that pregnant drug users are pregnant women first who have an additional problem with drugs. Their obstetric management should be based on standard principles, with management of their drug use a related, but separate issue.

Identifying drug users' pregnancies as high risk does not necessarily mean that 'high-tech' obstetrics is needed to manage them.

Pregnant women who use drugs are often afraid of encountering negative staff attitudes – hostile social workers, patronizing doctors and judgemental midwives. They have all heard about children of users being taken into care at birth. However, no one will condemn them more than themselves for using drugs in pregnancy and if we endorse the stereotypic picture of a drug user, we can add to the problem by giving unhelpful treatment. Women then stay away from the services, seemingly confirming the attitude that they are unfit.

Management by a multi-disciplinary team

Components that affect the outcome of a pregnancy are multi-factorial. Women who use drugs potentially have a whole range of other problems – housing, financial, nutritional, smoking and relationships with other people. All of these need to be addressed, and may be more important or urgent than their drug use. The GP should be involved, particularly if prescribing substitute drugs, even when the woman is an in-patient. The GP should have good links with the local midwives and obstetrician, as well as with relevant social services. The pregnant woman needs a key midwife, who should be a team member offering support and backup. The team should also include a health visitor and drug worker (if appropriate). All those involved need to be included at all stages.

Drug use by one or both parents does not by itself constitute neglect, abuse or a reason for registration of the child on the child protection register. Every local authority should have a written policy about drug-using parents and all professionals involved should be aware of the policy.[4] Confidentiality must be maintained at all times.

Management of antenatal care

Balancing stability of the drug-using woman with the lowest possible dose for the fetus

There are many myths surrounding the effects on the fetus of drugs in pregnancy, in part because there is a lack of good evidence and in part due to prejudice. There have also been theoretical concerns about dangers of antenatal detoxification but these have not been borne out in practice.[5]

Until recently, detoxification regimens during pregnancy have been rigid, slow and usually limited to the mid-trimester because of the perceived risk of miscarriage in the first, and premature labour in the third trimester. Maternal drug use has been considered incompatible with good parenting so although detoxification is discouraged during pregnancy, abstinence is considered essential after delivery!

Pregnancy is a time of change in any woman's life, and this can be used to promote behavioural change in drug use. Most women will want to reduce or stop their drug use during pregnancy but conversely there is a risk of relapse because of feelings of low self-esteem and anxieties about their parenting skills. While reduction in consumption of drugs during pregnancy to minimize fetal effects is important, this should not be at the expense of stability. The aim should be to help women decide on an individually appropriate approach to management.

The reduction in drugs taken during pregnancy can take place with the patient as an out-patient or as an in-patient. In-patient care tends to be more successful, allowing the woman time away from other struggles and distancing her from the drug supply. A stay in the antenatal ward facilitates monitoring of the pregnancy, and being with other pregnant women may provide a more positive experience than admission to a psychiatric ward.

Effects of drugs on the fetus and baby

Non-specific effects

Information about the precise effects of different drugs on the fetus is difficult to obtain and can be unreliable. Intra-uterine growth retardation and preterm deliveries contribute to increased rates of low birth-weight and consequently an increased perinatal mortality rate. These outcomes are however multifactorial and also affected by factors associated with socioeconomic deprivation, including smoking. The frequent association between deprivation and problem drug use makes precise causal relationships difficult to determine.

Problems in the baby are related to:

• gestation of pregnancy when drug is taken
• the route, quantity and duration of drug use

- pharmacology of the drug

- non-specific factors.[6]

Determining a safe level of drug use is not without problems. Data are poor since many studies are retrospective and rely on self-reporting of drug use, often some time after the event. Overall the presence and/or severity of neonatal withdrawal symptoms is dose related, although a close correlation does not exist for individual cases. Consequently, a woman's level of drug use cannot accurately predict the condition of the baby, neither will its condition accurately reflect the mother's level of drug use.

It is also known that many of the problems occur equally in babies born to non-drug using women in similar social conditions. In a sample of 200 pregnant drug-using women in Glasgow, less than 10% of babies were born before 37 weeks gestation, 12.5% had birth weights of <2.5 kg and 11% had birth weights <10th percentile. This was comparable to outcomes in non drug-using women from similar backgrounds.[7] However, ongoing study with a sample size now treble this suggests overall outcomes may be less favourable. Another study of 103 opiate-dependent women on prescribed methadone (of whom half were using additional illicit drugs) revealed no significant increase in antenatal complications in association with maternal drug use and highlighted the major contribution of smoking to low birth weight.[8]

With the exception of craniofacial abnormalities linked to alcohol consumption, and reports of an association between cleft palate and benzodiazepine use, maternal drug use does not appear to cause an increase in congenital abnormalities.

While significant drug use during pregnancy is undoubtedly associated with increased rates of still birth and neonatal death, the presence of other contributory social and lifestyle factors makes it difficult to attribute fetal deaths to drug use *per se*. There is evidence of an increase in the rate of sudden infant death.

Specific effects

Alcohol

Alcohol consumption during pregnancy causes similar non-specific effects and it can also cause developmental anomalies in the fetus.

However, there does not appear to be close correlation between dose or pattern of consumption and the presence of fetal alcohol syndrome.

Heroin, methadone and other opiates

Non-specific effects, such as low birth weight and prematurity occur in this group of drug users.

Benzodiazepines

Non-specific effects occur as with opiate use.

A link between cleft lip and palate and benzodiazepine use in early pregnancy has been noted, but is not conclusively proven.

Cocaine

Cocaine is a powerful vasoconstrictor and its use in pregnancy is associated with increased risks of abortion, placental abruption, intrauterine death and fetal hypoxia due to reduced placental blood flow. Binges of cocaine can potentially cause fetal brain infarcts due to reduced cerebral blood flow. In addition, it has been suggested that cocaine use during pregnancy may directly affect fetal neuronal development causing persistent neurobehavioral deficiencies, but a direct causal link is difficult to establish.[6]

Amphetamines and Ecstasy

These drugs tend to be used mostly on an occasional basis and specific problems have not been noted.

Reduction of drugs by the mother during pregnancy

- Reduction can occur at any speed and at any stage during pregnancy.

- Base on what the woman can tolerate or is willing to try.

- Should be woman directed and not doctor restricted.

Regimen for reducing opiates – methadone and heroin

The most appropriate regimen will depend on the severity of withdrawal symptoms, including sleep disturbance and the woman's ability to cope.

1   Just stopping 'cold turkey' can be an option with opiates, particularly heroin, because of its short half-life.

2   If this is not possible, establish a dose of methadone equivalent to the heroin or other opiate being used. Heroin may cause less withdrawal symptoms in the baby, but has the disadvantage that it cannot be taken by the oral route, has a short half-life so amounts therefore fluctuate and can only be prescribed by a psychiatrist with a heroin licence.

3   Some centres have found it helpful to divide the dose of methadone into a twice-daily schedule but this is inconsistent.

4   Try to convert all methadone to oral rather than injectable, as a harm-reduction procedure.

5   If starting on a high dose, the first half of the detoxification programme can usually occur at a faster rate.

6   When the woman has chosen to try as an out-patient, a reasonable regimen would be to reduce methadone by 5 mg every four to five days, according to the woman's response but this could be faster or slower.

7   As an in-patient on the antenatal ward, try reducing methadone more quickly, e.g. 5 mg every one or two days.

8   A partial detoxification may be a good compromise. At doses of 15 mg and below there are rarely any significant fetal effects.

9   If detoxification is unsuccessful and drug use becomes uncontrolled, the reduction could be stopped or the methadone increased until stability is regained, i.e. detoxification and maintenance can be interchanged.

Case history

Sally, aged 24 years, had been using diazepam from the age of 15, heroin since the age of 19 and methadone, supplied by her partner, for three years. She is 16 weeks pregnant and is sent to register with the GP by the midwife at the local hospital. She is using 150 mg of methadone and 30 mg of diazepam daily. She wants to be off all drugs by the time of the birth. She decides to try to reduce in the community. When she reaches 100 mg of methadone daily she requests a stay in hospital. She manages well and is discharged on 50 mg of methadone after two weeks. On re-entering the community she almost immediately relapses and starts to inject methadone ampoules. She again asks for help and has a further in-patient stay of over three weeks. She is discharged on no diazepam and 30 mg of methadone, which she reduces to 12 mg over the last few weeks of pregnancy. The baby is born without withdrawals and to date mother is coping well with the baby and using only 20 mg of methadone.

Regimen for reducing benzodiazepines

1   Just stopping may be risky for the woman because of the possibility of convulsions.

2   Benzodiazepines may cause long lasting and difficult to control withdrawal symptoms in the baby so any reduction in level of use is a bonus.

3   Convert all benzodiazepines to diazepam (see Chapter 8 for dose equivalents). A daily starting dose of 35–40 mg would be reasonable.

4   It is best to split the dose of diazepam into three roughly equal doses and reduce the doses in rotation, e.g. first the morning dose, then the mid-day dose, then the night dose.

5   During an in-patient stay, the dose can be reduced by 5 mg of diazepam every one to three days. Even with such a quick reduction no fits have been observed in many hundreds of women. Most women can be detoxified off diazepam in about a week with no ill-effects.

6 Out-patient reduction is not an option with which all specialists agree. If it is undertaken, the rate of reduction should be slower than for in-patients, say 5–10 mg per week, but again it should be decided according to the woman's ability to cope.

Case history

Doris, aged 26 years, had been registered at the practice for many years. She came from an extremely dysfunctional family, was sexually abused as a child, had two brothers die from overdoses and one who was a chronic alcoholic. The GP was prescribing 60 mg of methadone mixture and 60 mg of diazepam, although she used up to 120 mg of diazepam in binges. Diazepam was her first choice of drug. She had tried many detoxification programmes in the community and in residential units and had had some periods of abstinence. She presented with abdominal pain and was diagnosed as 14 weeks pregnant. She was using the contraceptive pill and condoms but remembered missing a few pills a couple of months ago when her partner had been absent intermittently. She wanted to be drug-free before the birth and immediately began to reduce her non-prescribed drug use. She then continued with a detoxification programme at home, until about 28 weeks gestation, when she requested further help. She was finding the diazepam reduction difficult and was admitted to the antenatal ward. Over the next seven weeks, with a combination of in- and out-patient treatment she reduced to 10 mg of methadone and 20 mg of diazepam. At 35 weeks, she went into spontaneous labour and delivered normally. The baby had some benzodiazepine withdrawals, which began after three days and required treatment with a small reducing dose of benzodiazepines for three days. Mother and baby were discharged together and continue to do well with a lot of support from their grandmother and their father's sister.

Regimen for reducing cocaine

1 Stopping cocaine altogether is the best option as there is no safe drug for substitute prescribing.

2 This may be helped by a short in-patient stay or by counselling or local self-help groups, such as Cocaine Anonymous.

Maternal health problems

Nutrition

Many women are poor and suffer social deprivation, as well as using drugs. Encouragement to eat a good diet is essential. Think about supplements, such as protein drinks, if the diet is inadequate. Weighing, although abandoned for most antenatal care schemes, can be a useful marker as to the stability of drug use.[5]

Anaemia

Iron deficiency tends to be commoner but treatment may exacerbate constipation already present because of drugs (especially methadone) or simply a poor diet.

Dental

Many drug users have bad teeth because of poor nutrition and poor personal hygiene, made worse by years of taking oral methadone. Pregnancy is a good time to address this problem. It is important to deal with bad teeth since these are a focus of infection which could represent a significant risk for women with a history of endocarditis and/or cardiac valvular disease. Remember that reducing analgesic drugs, such as heroin, may draw attention to the problem of toothache.

Infection

Complications from injecting such as abscesses can occur in pregnancy, increasing the need for fast-track admission of pregnant women into services. Stabilizing on oral drugs is safer than continued injecting of street drugs, which often have impurities that further damage the veins. Needle exchanges and/or provision of clean equipment are vital for women who continue to inject.

Hepatitis B

All pregnant women, drug users or not, should have their hepatitis B status checked and if not immune, drug using women should be offered a course of hepatitis B vaccine after delivery. Persistent carrier status is uncommon among those infected in adulthood. Over 50% of drug users have been found to be immune from a previous infection.[9] If the mother is hepatitis antigen-positive the baby should receive active immunization at birth and passive immunization by administration of immunoglobulin. If the mother is immune but not infectious, some would consider this a marker for a high-risk household and would advocate immunization of the baby.

Hepatitis C

Hepatitis C is a relatively newly identified virus (1990) and its effects on women and babies are still being investigated. Small surveys suggest as many as 75–80% of injecting drug users are positive for hepatitis C.[10] Some women will have non-specific symptoms of tiredness and lethargy, but many will not suffer symptoms until many years after infection. The disease itself rarely causes problems in pregnancy, except for non-specific effects. There is a low, possibly less than 10%, chance of hepatitis C being passed on to the baby. This chance is increased when there is co-infection with HIV. Hepatitis C appears to cause minimal problems in the neonate but the clinical picture is not yet clear.

HIV

Pregnancy seems to have no adverse effect on women who are HIV positive unless they are significantly immunocompromised, in which case it may cause further deterioration. There is no adverse effect on pregnancy outcome.[11] The main concern is vertical transmission of infection to the fetus. Transmission can occur at any stage of pregnancy although the majority are at the time of delivery. A number of interventions are available to reduce the likelihood of transmission at each stage. However, none of these interventions can eliminate risk. All women should be given information to enable them to make appropriate choices about antenatal testing and obstetric management.

It is important to remember that:

• pregnant women need to be given full information about blood-borne viruses and screening tests

- women must be allowed to make their own choices

- women's choices may be different from those of the health carers.

Case history

Jill, aged 25 years, had been injecting drugs over many years. She had been known to be HIV positive for five years and had recently begun to develop symptoms, with skin rashes, anaemia, low platelets and chest infections. She was receiving a very large injectable script of methadone, dexedrine and diazepam from a private prescriber. She became pregnant by a man who had been a patient of the surgery for many years. He requested help for her. During pregnancy she changed to oral methadone at a smaller dose, stopped all cocaine and amphetamines and reduced her benzodiazepines. She did not want to stop altogether. Her reduction was helped by a period of respite care in the local HIV hospice. She was given all the information about possible options and decided to opt for delivery by section and not to breastfeed. She had been given AZT several years before and had been very unwell when taking it so had ceased after three months. All tests indicated that the baby was not infected with HIV.

Management of labour

This is similar to any other woman, but pain relief needs special attention. More opiates may not be helpful if all the receptors are full. There should be a low threshold for offering an epidural. There may be increased placental insufficiency in pregnancies of drug using women leading to an increased risk of intrapartum hypoxia, fetal distress and meconium staining.

Postnatal care

It is easy to forget the mother's needs at this stage, especially if the baby is experiencing withdrawal symptoms, although this may be the very time she needs more support. If the baby is withdrawing, the mother may have difficulty bonding with it. She must be reassured that it is not a failure of her mothering skills. The professionals involved must not transmit feelings of blame to the mother, even if they are involved in the care of her sick baby.

Contraception

Discussions about what contraception to use should commence early in pregnancy. Always recommend the use of condoms for prevention of infections, even when another method of contraception has also been chosen.

Breastfeeding

Breastfeeding should be encouraged, even if the mother is continuing to use drugs. The possible exceptions are if she is HIV positive (because of the doubling of the HIV transfer rate when breastfeeding), or hepatitis C positive, because of the uncertainty around hepatitis C. Very small amounts of the drugs she is taking will pass across in the breast milk, matching exactly the combination of drugs the baby received in utero. This will help reduce the withdrawals and can diminish the need for treatment of the baby.

The neonate

Mother and baby need to be treated as a unit. Withdrawal symptoms in the neonate may occur if the mother has been regularly taking illicit or substitute drugs, such as methadone, but can also result from occasional drug use in the mother. The greater the reduction achieved during pregnancy, the smaller the number of babies who will experience withdrawals.[7]

Signs of withdrawal are vague and multiple and tend to occur within 48–72 hours of delivery if the mother continued using up to delivery.[8] They include a spectrum of symptoms: excessive wakefulness, restlessness and irritability, often with scratching, high-pitched cry, hunger but with ineffective sucking, sneezing, stuffy nose and salivation. Sweating and dehydration, tremors, vomiting and diarrhoea, hyperthermia (>38°C) and tachypnoea (>60 per minute), yawning, hiccups and fist-sucking can occur. The other end of the spectrum include hypertonicity and convulsions but these are not common.

The baby should be returned to the postnatal ward with the mother shortly after delivery. The mother should be asked to monitor the baby for signs of withdrawal. She should attend to all the baby's needs and involve the midwives if she needs help or is unsure. The baby should be transferred to the neonatal unit if there is significant cerebral irritation with the risk of fitting, and/or excessive weight loss due to poor feeding.

Every woman should meet the paediatrician during pregnancy and have possible outcomes explained to her. She should also be shown round the neonatal unit during pregnancy, so it is familiar territory if her baby needs to be transferred there after birth.

The most appropriate drugs for treatment of withdrawal symptoms in neonates are still a matter of debate. Treatment can be either symptomatic or by substitution therapy. Phenobarbitone can be used as a stat. dose, with an option to continue for one or two days. If the baby does not settle, chlorpromazine can be tried. Evidence from the USA suggests that methadone is an appropriate drug to use, particularly if this has been used by the mother.[8] Babies born to mothers who have been using benzodiazepines in pregnancy may take longer to settle. If withdrawal symptoms continue this may suggest organic damage.

Social factors

Socioeconomic deprivation is associated with less effective use of health care services and this may be even more marked when there is associated drug use. As in the case of non drug-using women, poor attendance for antenatal care is not indicative of a lack of parental concern. Outcomes of pregnancies are often worse in women who do not attend antenatal care regardless of whether they use drugs or not since non-attendance may be indicative of chaotic lifestyle, chaotic drug use or other social problem. Research shows no deep gulf between drug-using and non drug-using mothers in terms of attitudes.[12] These women have the same concerns for and pride in their present and forthcoming children.

Because of the range of problems, women need to be managed in the context of their family and background by a multi-disciplinary team who are all working with common aims and philosophy.

Drug use *per se* should never be a reason for taking a child into care. Child care abilities should be assessed on the basis of stability of lifestyle and levels of harmful behaviour. Planning for delivery and after-care needs to start in pregnancy and involve the parents, social services and all relevant health care professions namely obstetricians, midwifes, paediatricians, GP and health visitor.

Before the birth

A planning meeting (not a case conference) called by the social work department needs to take place in the second half of pregnancy. Here, all professionals can meet with the parent/s to identify problems, set goals and plan support networks. A formal case conference is only necessary if there are significant concerns that the parent/s may not be able to cope. A full explanation of the purpose of this meeting should be given to the parent/s so she/they can be involved to the extent they choose.

The social services department from the area where the woman lives should take responsibility for the planning and be involved before the birth. A named social worker, whom the woman can build a relationship with is preferable.

After the birth

The social worker, who is already familiar with the woman and her family, provides continuity after birth. This may be a very stressful time for the mother, particularly if the baby is transferred to the neonatal unit. She may also have problems with housing and finances, and may welcome help and support with these problems if not already resolved during pregnancy. The woman and her partner may also wish to know about possible treatment options including residential rehabilitation. There are, however, very few residential rehabilitation units that will take children together with their mother and/or father, and the ones that do have extremely long waiting lists. Funding can be difficult. There may be possibilities for treatment on a day care basis.

Long-term development problems reported by some to affect babies of drug-using women are multifactorial. A five-year follow-up study in Holland reported an increased incidence of health problems and abnormalities of physical, mental and behavioural development among children born to drug-using women.[13] It is impossible to determine the precise contribution of the various possible aetiological factors including maternal drug use *per se* and such findings are inconsistently reported.

Summary

Pregnant drug-using women should have access to and be encouraged to use appropriate effective, non-judgemental services provided by a multi-disciplinary team. Such services should deal with all her problems and her drug use should be managed in the context of her other social problems. Stability of drug use and consequently stability of lifestyle should be the objective rather than abstinence. Women should be involved in decisions about their management which should aim to reduce drug use to the lowest dose compatible with reasonable stability. This balance may alter once the baby is born and minimization of neonatal withdrawal symptoms is no longer an issue. The level of substitution therapy may need to be increased post-natally.

All drug-using women should be provided with ongoing care and support. A collaborative approach from the relevant services is essential to enable such women to cope with the demands of parenting against the background of multiple social problems.

11

Young people and drugs
Julian Cohen

Trends in drug use by young people

Drugs are a normal part of every child's life. Nearly every young child has taken a range of medicines and many are regular consumers of caffeine in soft drinks, some confectionery, tea and coffee. Research also shows that even young children are aware of legal and illegal drugs, to an extent that often surprises their parents and teachers.[1]

Alcohol is the most popular drug of choice amongst young people. Surveys have shown that over 95% of 15–16 year olds have had an alcoholic drink, that about 70% of 13–17 year olds have brought alcohol from a pub or off-licence and that about one third of 13–16 year olds drink alcohol at least once a week.[2,3] In the late teens and early twenties alcohol consumption is about 50% above the adult average and there is a higher prevalence of heavy drinking and drunkenness than at any other age. There has been a recent trend towards consumption of drinks with high-alcohol content, especially strong lagers and ciders, and of alcoholic lemonades and other 'alco-pop' drinks. Whilst overall alcohol consumption among young people has not been rising, this latter development may signal an increase amongst younger age groups who previously have been deterred by the taste of alcohol.

Cigarette smoking has been declining in the adult population but this has not been the case amongst young people. Recent surveys show that about 5% of 13 year olds smoke regularly, rising to 20–30% by the age of 15 and almost one third by later teens.[4] More young females than young males now smoke cigarettes. The only growth market for tobacco companies is amongst young, particularly working-class, women.

Use of illicit drugs

More young people are experimenting with illegal and socially unacceptable drugs compared with a few years ago and they are starting at a younger age. Recent local studies, carried out in urban and
rural areas, show a third to a half of 15–16 year olds have used an
illegal drug at least once.[5,6] According to the Institute for the Study of
Drug Dependence 'The relatively stable youth drug use patterns of
the mid-80s were disturbed in the late 80s and ... by the 90s there
was increased use of established drugs like cannabis, solvents, amphetamine and magic mushrooms and an upsurge in use of ecstasy
and LSD'.[7]

A survey of teenagers in the North-West of England found few
differences in drug-using patterns between working-class, inner-city
young people and those from middle-class, 'leafy' suburbs.[8] The survey also found little difference between girls and boys and between
black and white youngsters, although use was less in youngsters of
Asian origin. Many of the young people may have used illegal drugs
only once or occasionally but over 20% of the total sample were
classed as regular users, particularly of cannabis. Other illegal drugs
were more likely to be used on an occasional basis.

Solvents and young people

Solvent use is not new but hit the headlines in the 1980s especially in the form of 'glue sniffing'. Since then the trend has been
away from glue towards aerosols and butane gas, and occasionally other solvent-based products. Solvent use tends to occur
amongst younger age groups.

Deaths associated with solvent use have declined in recent
years, from over 150 a year, to under 70. Recent anecdotal
evidence suggests that solvent use has declined in fashion in the
mid-1990s, possibly in part as a consequence of widespread
availability of drugs such as cannabis.

Surveys also show that the number of young people who have used
drugs increases in the post-16 age group and that 'dance drugs' such
as Ecstasy and amphetamine are particularly popular. Some com-
mentators have suggested that there may be over 500 000 mainly
young people using Ecstasy during any one weekend.

The Health Education Authority has released preliminary results from a survey of almost 5000 11–35 year olds in England conducted in late 1995.[9] Of the total sample, 70% had been offered illegal drugs and 45% had tried at least one illegal drug at some time in their life. 15% had used a drug during the last month. The survey results are shown in Table 11.1.

Table 11.1: Survey results for illegal drug use[9]

Age (years)	Ever offered %	Ever used %	Used during past month %
11–14	25	6	2
14–16	62	30	13
16–19	82	55	27
20–22	86	62	26
23–25	80	54	18
26–30	70	45	15
31–35	64	42	8

Use of illicit drugs was most prevalent in the 16–19 and 20–22 age groups. The survey results show the recent increase in young people's drug use in that fewer 26–35 year olds had ever been offered or used drugs than in the 16–25 age groups. However, the high figures for the older age groups also demonstrate that such drug use is not a new phenomenon.

Surveys conducted in Scotland show similar trends to those carried out in England and Wales although there may be evidence for suggesting that illicit drug use is slightly higher amongst young people in Scotland and that temazepam use is more prevalent than south of the border.[10,11]

'New' drugs

Ecstasy was first used on a widespread basis in the UK in 1988, despite the fact that it has been in existence since the early 1900s. LSD took off in this country in the 1960s and its popularity waned in the 1970s, only to become widely used again in the late 1980s and 1990s. The last couple of years have seen use of 'new' drugs amongst young people, such as GHB, ketamine, certain Ecstasy-like substances and various 'legal highs', often made from herbal mixtures. Different drugs come

continued

into, and go out of, fashion. Some take off in a big way and become established. Others hit the headlines but do not become used on a wide scale. The later part of the 1990s is likely to see new, designer drugs come on to the scene, often accompanied by new media drug scares.

Steroids

Use of anabolic steroids and other performance-enhancing drugs has become much more common in recent years, especially amongst people who are committed to sports and body building. There is also evidence that some young people take steroids in an attempt to improve their looks on the dance floor. Steroids can be taken orally and are also injected. Steroids are often available through gyms and health clubs and many local drug services who operate needle exchange schemes have significant numbers of steroid-using clients.

Cocaine tends to be expensive and outside the price range of most younger people. Crack, a form of cocaine, is not widely available and despite media scares is mainly focused on certain inner-city areas. Heroin use is still widespread and although there have been recent reports of a resurgence in use amongst young people it still tends to be mostly used by disenfranchized young people living in deprived areas. Most dependent heroin users are in the 20–30-year-old age group. Non-medical use of benzodiazepines, especially temazepam, has also increased in recent years. Some dependent opiate users prepare temazepam for injection and this has caused problems in some areas, particularly in Scotland. Some young people also smoke heroin or take tranquillizers to soften the 'come down' from regular use of drugs, such as Ecstasy and amphetamine.

In summary, use of both illegal and other socially unacceptable drugs is becoming much more common amongst young people. There is talk of the 'normalization' of young people's drug use, whereby use of drugs such as cannabis, LSD, amphetamine, 'poppers' and Ecstasy has become integrated into youth culture and is not seen as a 'big deal' by the young people themselves, whatever adults may think of it. Much drug use amongst young people is of an experimental and occasional nature. Many teenagers also now use drugs like cannabis and 'dance drugs' in a regular, relatively controlled, recreational way much as many adults use alcohol. Only a small percentage use drugs in a very chaotic or dependent way, or inject.

Patterns of drug use vary in different parts of the country. In some areas, prevalence of drug use is particularly high and drug dealing and associated criminal activity is very blatant. In other areas drug use and dealing may be more low key. Despite local variations it is clear that young people's drug use occurs in all communities, social classes and ethnic groups and that female use has caught up with that by males. Many young people cease regular use of illegal drugs by their mid-20s as they taken on adult responsibilities. However, the adverse economic outlook means fewer young people achieve stability by this age (in terms of employment, housing, relationships, having children etc.) and points to a possible elongation of illicit drug careers and an increase in the number of young, dependent users.[12]

Problems associated with young people's drug use

The vast majority of people who use drugs come to no harm, and many will feel that they have benefited (and may well have done so) from the relaxation, diversion or temporarily improved social, intellectual or physical performance that can be afforded by some drugs. But there are serious risks....[13]

Drug effects and risks are the result of interaction between three factors.

1   *Drug factors* – everything connected with the substance itself and how it is taken.

2   *The set* – factors concerning the person using drugs, especially their physical and mental health.

3   *The setting* – what users are doing at the time, where they are and who they are with.

Drug factors

Different drugs carry different risks as the following examples illustrate.

•   *Alcohol, heroin and tranquillizers* – these drugs can lead to physical dependence if they are taken regularly.

- *Amphetamine, cocaine, crack (a form of cocaine) and Ecstasy* – these drugs are strong 'uppers' (stimulants) and can be particularly dangerous to people who have heart or blood pressure problems.

- *Alcohol, heroin and tranquillizers* – these drugs are 'downers' (depressants) and taken in large quantities or combination can lead to fatal overdose.

- *LSD and magic mushrooms (and to a lesser extent strong forms of cannabis and Ecstasy)* – these drugs are hallucinogenic and users may become very disturbed and do dangerous things especially if they are already anxious or depressed.

The risks of drug use also vary with the following.

- How strong the dose is of the drug that is taken.

- How often it is taken.

- What else might be mixed with it. Many illegal powders and tablets are adulterated and have all sorts of contaminants mixed with them, such as chalk, talcum powder, brick dust, etc.

- Whether different drugs are taken together. Young people may be under the influence of more than one drug at any one time.

- How a drug is taken. Injecting tends to be the most dangerous drug-taking method, although there have been many method-specific deaths with solvent use when, for example, young people have squirted butane or aerosols straight down the throat or suffocated by placing the head inside plastic bags.

The set

Drug risks also vary depending on the following.

- *Physical health* – heart and blood pressure problems, asthma, diabetes, epilepsy and liver problems can make drug use more dangerous.

- *Mental health* – people who are anxious or depressed often find drug use makes them feel worse and could lead to them endangering themselves or others. They are more likely to use drugs in a dependent way as an attempt to block out unpleasant feelings about themselves, others and the world around them.

- *Body weight* – lighter people find the same amount of drug affects them more than a heavier person. People with eating disorders can also find drug use makes their condition worse. This may be a particular issue for young women who use amphetamine or Ecstasy and smoke cigarettes.

- *Lack of knowledge and experience* – a person new to drug use may be unsure what to expect or do, may feel anxious and be more likely to get into problems. A small quantity of drug may be more likely to have a large effect.

- *Gender* – drug use can affect males and females differently because of different body weight and physical make up and the different expectations of males and females.

The setting

Where people are and what they are doing whilst on drugs can also have a bearing on the risks involved. Examples include the following.

- Taking drugs in dangerous, out of the way environments. Some youngsters use drugs near river banks, main roads or railway lines or in derelict buildings. This increases the likelihood of accidents and means help is not easily at hand if needed.

- Driving a car or bike or operating machinery whilst under the influence of alcohol or other drugs. Again accidents are more likely.

- Use of Ecstasy in crowded, hot clubs and dancing for hours without stopping has led to over 70 deaths since 1988 from overheating and dehydration.

- Being in sexual situations whilst under the influence of drugs may increase the likelihood of people having sex when they are not sure they want to and makes it more difficult to practise safer sex and use condoms if they do have intercourse.

Young people may experience physical or mental health problems as a result of drug use. They may also experience related lifestyle problems involving changes in friendships and family relationships, poor school, college or work performance, financial problems, criminal behaviour and associations, getting into trouble with the police and conflict with parents/carers. Young people's drug use creates problems for families and the wider community but some of these problems may also be to do with how adults respond to young people in general, rather than to the drug user specifically.

Young people may also experience problems because of use of drugs by other people, especially parents/carers, brothers and sisters, other family members and their friends.

'Risks' and 'problems' may be perceived very differently by young people and adults. Young people may sometimes see risk as attractive. Adults are often very selective about their perceptions of risk and encourage young people to be involved in other risky activities, such as outdoor pursuits. Young people may also not see drug-related problems as being of much significance or may enjoy status and attention from experiencing them. Parents or teachers may see any contact with drugs as a problem whilst the young person concerned may see their drug use as a pleasure.

When considering drug problems it is important to assess risk realistically and when there are problems to ask what exactly they are, who they are a problem for and how the young person involved feels about them.

Drug-related deaths

Deaths from illegal drug use tend to be exaggerated whilst deaths from use of tobacco and alcohol are often glossed over. Each year in the UK over 110 000 people die prematurely from tobacco-related diseases. Estimates of alcohol-related deaths vary from 15 000–30 000 per annum. Many alcohol-related fatal overdoses and accidents involve young people. Deaths associated with solvent use have been between 70 and 150 young people each year and the total number of deaths associated with illegal drug use in people of all ages in the UK was recorded as 1620 in 1994.[6]

Response to young people's drug use

Much of the response to young people's drug use had been in the realms of a 'moral panic'. Politicians and the tabloid media see drug use as wrong and in need of stamping out. Fear, ignorance, scare-mongering and exaggeration have been all too common. One result has been 'deviancy amplification', whereby there is very little open dialogue between young people and adult society.[14]

The main responses to young people's drug use have been in terms of control, care and education. Attempts at control have included legal measures, such as developments in policing and detection, moves towards more cautioning for possession of illicit drugs and stiffer penalties for dealing and trafficking. For young people control measures have also led to a significant increase in school and college expulsions.

Traditional drug services, with their emphasis on heroin injectors, methadone prescribing and needle exchanges have, in the main, failed to attract younger users who are unlikely to see themselves as 'addicts'.[15] A few agencies are now beginning to provide services for young drug users and for parents who are concerned about their children's use. This has included diversification of traditional services, the setting up of dedicated drug services for young people and parents and the integration of drug issues within generic youth counselling and advice services.

Education and information programmes have mainly been initiated through the media and schools. Historically such programmes have focused on primary prevention – attempting to stop young people using drugs – on the assumption that users are deficient in knowledge of drugs, skills to resist peer pressure or self-esteem. However, evaluations of primary prevention programmes have shown them to be ineffective in preventing drug use and to be based on fallacious assumptions.[16,17] Whilst the government and statutory bodies have tended to ignore this research evidence, more local programmes are now being based on education and harm reduction principles – providing accurate and balanced information and encouraging young people to think and act for themselves – rather than more propagandist campaigns.[18]

The role of general practice

Traditional drug services rarely cater for younger drug users and their parents. The fact that most younger people and parents already use GPs means that general practice can play an important role in responding to drug problems amongst the younger age group. This might include the following.

- Providing accurate information about drug use and services available. This can include displaying posters, provision of leaflets and providing information by word of mouth.

- Sensitively exploring issues around possible drug use when young people consult for other reasons.

- Counselling young drug users and family members.

- Appropriate prescribing of medication to young drug users. This might be medication to alleviate withdrawal symptoms or the occasional prescribing of substitute drugs for young dependent users. GPs should also try to avoid prescribing potentially addictive drugs, such as benzodiazepines, to young people.

- Helping young drug users optimize their physical health by monitoring and giving advice about weight, nutrition, sexual health, etc.

- Referral to dedicated drug services where appropriate.

- Provision of support and advice to community-based health workers.

- Involvement in multi-disciplinary networks to develop working relationships with other agencies and influence the provision of local services.

In the past, general practice has tended to focus on prescribing substitute drugs for older opiate users and many practices have been mistrustful of drug users and reluctant to deal with them sensitively.[19] Work with younger drug users and parents needs to go beyond a 'medical model'. In particular, young people and parents will need to feel that GPs and practice staff are approachable, non-judgemental and non-patronising. As with contraception services confidentiality will be important to young people. Parents will often need reassurance and support in understanding and helping their children. To be able to perform these roles members of the practice team will need access to up-to-date drug information as well as training and support.

12

Practical aspects of managing drug users

Judy Bury

The DoH document *Drug Misuse and Dependence: Guidelines on Clinical Management* published in 1991[1] offered 'flexible guidance to help all doctors, within the context of their own clinical practice, to provide an effective response to patients with problems of drug misuse'. The guidelines restated the view, expressed in various government publications since the mid-1980s, that 'the GP is in a specially favourable position to understand a patient's drug problem', but went on to acknowledge that 'the GP needs to strike a balance between making help readily accessible to those in urgent need while maintaining appropriate vigilance to avoid abuse of the service'.[1]

In 1993 a report from the ACMD,[2] while emphasizing the central role of GPs once again, acknowledged that there was little evidence of a significant increase in the number of GPs becoming involved. Many GPs are willing to work with drug users but may become disillusioned by a sense of failure or because of problems that drug users sometimes cause for the practice. They may feel untrained and uncertain about how to deal with patients who can be very challenging. This chapter deals with some practical aspects of caring for drug users in general practice.

Implications for the practice

Caring for drug users in general practice can cause problems for the primary care team and disruption to the running of the practice.

- Drug users can be difficult and demanding, and working with them can be stressful.

- Caring for drug users may cause disagreements between individual doctors and between doctors and other staff.

- Staff and other patients may be upset by the behaviour of some drug users.

Many of these problems can be reduced by finding a balance between offering compassionate care and setting limits to behaviour.

The principles outlined can also be useful in other situations in general practice, for example the patient who repeatedly requests inappropriate home visits, or the patient who is reluctant to stop hypnotics.

Setting limits to behaviour: the use of practice policies and agreements

Doctor A has been working with drug users for six years but does not feel he is getting anywhere. He fears he has been conned and worries that drugs prescribed by him are being sold on the street. His partners think he is too soft with drug users and object to seeing his patients when he goes on holiday. On returning from holiday he finds that four of his drug-using patients have been put off the practice list in his absence. This leads to discussions within the practice about establishing a practice policy for dealing with drug users. Doctor A is encouraged to apply firmer limits to the behaviour of his drug-using patients, while the other doctors agree to become more involved and to discuss the management of difficult patients rather than automatically putting them off the list.

Some GPs are reluctant to apply firm limits to the behaviour of drug users, believing that to do so would damage the doctor–patient relationship. In fact, this is far from being the case. Drug users have often lacked parenting, or at least appropriate parenting, and may be stuck in adolescent behaviour. In order to mature they need care and concern on the one hand, and firm and consistent boundaries on the other. In order to provide such boundaries, practices benefit from an agreed written policy about working with drug users. GPs should consider using agreements with drug users so that they are made aware of the policies of the practice and can be reminded of them when they forget. When drug users break the agreement, the appropriate sanction (e.g. warning, withdrawal of prescription, removal from list) should be applied consistently. Using such policies and agreements and applying sanctions in a consistent manner reduces the disruption caused by drug users to the running of a practice. It may also be beneficial for the drug user as it encourages maturation.

Practice policies

It is helpful for GPs in a practice to agree on certain aspects of working with drug users, or to agree to disagree. For example, in some practices all the GPs may be willing to see and/or prescribe for drug users whilst in others it may be agreed that only some of the GPs will do this work. It is always helpful for each drug user to see only a named GP (and a named deputy in his or her absence) to encourage continuity of care and to discourage shopping around between different GPs in the practice. The practice may wish to decide on policies relating to appointments, prescriptions and medication, and to define what it considers to be acceptable and unacceptable behaviour. These can then be written down and reviewed from time to time. There are many different kinds of practice policy – it is for each practice to decide on what seems appropriate and then to be consistent in its application.

It is useful to involve practice staff in discussions about the formulation of a practice policy. At the very least, once the practice policy has been agreed between the doctors, it is important to discuss it with any practice staff who might be involved in its implementation, especially receptionists, so that they are familiar with it and can raise any concerns about its application.

Issues to consider when formulating a practice policy

Appointments

- Is there a wish to have a named doctor for each drug user?
- Is there a policy about:
  - patients arriving without an appointment?
  - patients arriving late for an appointment?
  - patients asking for house calls to discuss medication?

Prescriptions and medication

- What is the policy on:
  - replacing lost prescriptions?
  - replacing lost medication?
  - releasing medication early?

Behaviour

- What is the practice attitude to drug users attending appointments accompanied by groups of friends?
- What action should be taken in the event of:
  - patients shouting at receptionists, or other patients?
  - patients threatening receptionists or other patients?
  - patients being violent?
- What are the situations in which the receptionist:
  - should call a doctor?
  - should call the police?
- Have the GPs agreed how they will respond to a call from a receptionist?

The importance of consistency

The receptionists in practice B have been encouraged to be firm with drug users. Drug users have been told that they will not be seen without an appointment. A drug user is demanding to be seen and the receptionist has stated clearly that he has to make an appointment. The drug user continues to demand to be seen. A GP comes out of her room, approaches the reception desk and invites the drug user into her room. The drug user emerges five minutes later holding a prescription which he waves triumphantly at the receptionist who feels undermined and put down.

Once a practice policy has been agreed it is important to be consistent in its application. If receptionists are expected to be firm in their application of the policy, it is important that they are supported. If a receptionist is interpreting the policy inappropriately, this should be discussed with him or her after the event, preferably involving the practice manager. If the policy is found to be inappropriate (for example, it may emerge that there are occasions when drug users can be seen without an appointment) then the policy should be reviewed and, if necessary, changed.

In the above scenario, familiar in most practices working with drug users, if the receptionist was interpreting the policy correctly, yet the GP felt that she had to intervene, perhaps to avoid distress to other patients, she could back up the receptionist by approaching the patient and reinforcing what the receptionist has said, e.g. 'Now, you know you can't be seen without an appointment, so let's see when the next appointment is available'. Alternatively, the GP can take the patient to her room to reinforce this message. (Some practices have a 'hassle' room – perhaps an interview room or an area off the waiting room – where upset, angry or disruptive patients can be dealt with away from public view in the waiting area). In either case, it is important for the GP to talk to the receptionist afterwards to support her in what she was doing and to explain what actions she has taken and why; e.g. 'You were handling that fine; I just came to bail you out because the noise was beginning to disturb other people; you'll be pleased to know that I reinforced what you were saying and sent him away without a prescription'.

Breaking and reviewing practice policies

Inevitably, even with the most clear cut policy, there will be occasions when a GP feels that the situation warrants contravening practice policy. Unexpected events, such as family bereavements, may necessitate prescriptions being issued early or without an appointment. It would obviously be insensitive and inappropriate for the GP to apply the policy rigidly in all circumstances. The term 'flexible rigidity' describes the approach that works best.

If a doctor feels that there are reasons why it is necessary to break the practice policy and give a patient a prescription without an appointment, it is important that he or she goes back to the receptionist afterwards to explain the reason for this.

Some practices find it helpful to have a forum for GPs to share with one another occasions on which they have found it necessary to go against the policy. This then allows the GPs to recognize that there are certain drug users who are regularly persuading them to bend the rules and/or if there are one or more GPs who find it difficult to apply the policy. It is also important to review the policy itself from time to time (perhaps twice a year) and involve all the staff in a discussion about how the policy is working.

Learning to say 'no'

> A drug user is consulting doctor C about a long-standing drug problem. She has run out of her prescribed drugs before her next prescription is due. The GP has refused to issue the prescription early but the drug user continues to ask for her drugs. For a while the GP continues to state that he will not give her the prescription but, as she continues to ask, the GP's resolve weakens and he says 'Well, all right then, just this once' and writes out the prescription.

There is no doubt that some GPs find it difficult to say 'no' to patients. They may find this particularly difficult if they have built up a relationship with a troublesome patient over a period of time and have persuaded themselves that it is appropriate to prescribe out of compassion and concern for their patient. It is important for a GP to know that giving into a patient is often not helpful. Just as with an adolescent, it can be quite undermining and unsettling for the patient if no limits are applied to his or her behaviour. Sometimes a GP starts by saying 'no' but, as in the scenario above, gives in after a while. Unfortunately, this may give the message to patients that if they nag for long enough then they will get what they want. If a GP is able to say 'no' and stick to this, the drug user may verbally abuse the GP at the time but will ultimately benefit from this application of limits. The drug user may even return and thank the doctor for his or her firmness.

Just as firmness without care and concern are unlikely to be helpful to the drug user, so care and concern without firmness are unlikely to be helpful either. Firmness also has the added advantage that it is likely to contribute to the smooth running of the practice.

This approach may be appropriate for a range of patients apart from drug users. By employing it with drug users, GPs may increase their confidence in applying it with other patients. Involving staff members in taking a team approach to working with drug users can enhance the working of the practice team. Thus, learning to work effectively with drug users can bring benefits to the practice as a whole.

Agreements or contracts

Once a practice policy has been agreed, an agreement or contract for the individual drug user can be drawn up to explain the policy of the practice with regard to appointments and prescriptions and to set out guidelines for the drug user about appropriate and inappropriate behaviour. As with policies, there are different types of agreement, and their contents will depend on the particular circumstances of the practice and the policy that has been agreed. It is helpful, however, if the agreement indicates what sanctions will be applied if the agreement is broken, and if these sanctions are not too specific. Thus, it is more helpful if the agreement says 'your prescriptions *may* be stopped' or 'you *may* be removed from the practice list' rather than 'you *will* be ...', thus allowing for a degree of flexibility. It is, however, useful to indicate if there are any 'absolute' offences, where flexibility will not be exercised. For example, a practice may decide that any violence to a receptionist or GP or to other patients, or any theft of prescriptions or prescription pads will always result in removal from the list. If so, this should be indicated in the agreement.

Some practices have found it helpful to think in terms of – and to explain the situation to the drug user in terms of – 'yellow card' and 'red card' offences, as in football. Thus, the breaking of some rules, such as repeatedly being late for appointments, might lead to a warning – a 'yellow card' – but if the drug user continues to break these rules in spite of the warning, then a 'red card' might apply, that is, the prescription may be stopped. Certain behaviour, such as violence or theft, may lead to an immediate 'red card', that is stopping the prescription or removal from the practice list.

Using agreements in the practice

> Two drug users are sitting in the waiting room of practice D. One is obviously intoxicated and from time to time shouts at the receptionist asking how much longer she must wait. The other is accompanied by a group of friends, some of whom are addressing other patients and using bad language.

It is simpler to have a standard agreement to which extra clauses can be added than to write out an agreement from scratch with each drug user. If a standard agreement is used, then the receptionists can be made aware of who is on an agreement. This can be very helpful to them in enforcing rules about certain aspects of behaviour. Thus the receptionist can say to a drug user 'You know that your medication can't be replaced' or, as in the above scenario, 'You know that you're not meant to come with lots of friends. I'm afraid they'll have to wait outside'.

The terms of the agreement can be discussed when the drug user is started on a prescription. This provides an opportunity for the drug user to ask questions, clarify any uncertainties and indicate whether they feel that the terms of the agreement are reasonable. The drug user can then be asked to sign the agreement, which is also signed by the doctor. A copy can be kept in the notes and a copy given to the patient. It can be referred back to in the future and the drug user reminded of its contents, especially if problems arise. Using an agreement in this way can encourage adult behaviour.

An example of an agreement is given below. A version of this is in use in a number of practices and practices are encouraged to adapt it for their own use.

Example of a patient agreement

Name .... Date ....

Doctors, staff and many patients have been upset by the behaviour of some surgery attenders. Many of these people are attending for prescriptions of addictive drugs. You are now receiving a regular prescription for addictive medication and we require you to accept these rules.

Behaviour

1 I agree to attend appointments promptly and quietly.

2 I agree not to upset the receptionists or other patients in the waiting room.

3 Due to restriction of space in the waiting room I agree to attend my appointments unaccompanied whenever possible.

Behaviour outside these limits may result in the receptionists or doctors asking you to leave the surgery premises. If necessary the police will be called and you may be removed from the practice list and no longer be seen at this surgery.

Prescription, medication and appointment

1 I agree to be responsible for making my appointments and checking that my appointment is correct in the appointment book.

2 I accept responsibility for turning up for my appointment on time.

3 I agree to attend only the doctors mentioned below, on this form, and to discuss my prescription only with them.

4 I agree not to use emergency appointments or house calls to discuss my prescription.

5 I agree to be responsible for my prescription and medication and recognize that these cannot be replaced.

6 I agree that no alteration will be made to my prescription without my own doctor's permission.

My doctor is Dr .... his/her half-day is ....

In his/her absence I will consult Dr ....

I HAVE READ THE ABOVE RULES, I UNDERSTAND WHAT THEY MEAN, I AGREE TO ABIDE BY THEM AND REALIZE THAT IF I DO NOT, MY PRESCRIPTION MAY BE STOPPED AND THAT I MAY BE REMOVED FROM THE DOCTOR'S MEDICAL LIST.

Signature .... (Patient) Date ....

Signature .... (Doctor) Date ....

Some practical hints

Apart from the use of policies and agreements, there are other practical points that can assist in the management of drug users in general
practice.

Appointments

Many unemployed drug users are semi-nocturnal, staying awake until
early morning and sleeping late. Early appointments are unlikely to
be kept. Care by receptionists in ensuring that they and the patient
have correctly noted the appointment time may save later confronta-
tion. The use of cards as in hospital out-patient departments is found
helpful by some practices.

Behaviour

The use of an 'incident book' for receptionists to record details of
patients behaving in a disruptive manner may serve both as a verbal
warning and as a way of assessing problems encountered. Sometimes
simply opening the book and asking for the patient's name can be
enough to defuse the situation – perhaps because the drug user is
reminded of school.

Although, in theory, putting a 'glass' panel between the receptionists and patients increases the receptionists' sense of security, many
practices have found that the behaviour of patients improves if such
panels are removed. Behaviour often also improves if the waiting area
is enlarged or made brighter.

Practices might want to consider the installation of panic buttons
in the reception area and/or in surgeries. If installed, it is essential
that GPs and staff are all clear about what action to take in the event
that the alarm is activated.

Many drug users are sensitive to the actual or perceived attitudes
of reception staff towards them. Treated with courtesy and considera-
tion, most will respond in kind.

Drug-user clinics

General practitioners may wish to consider seeing all or some of their
drug-using patients at a special clinic session. The main advantage of

this approach is that drug users are not mixing with and potentially upsetting other patients in the waiting room and that the doctor can work in collaboration with a drug counsellor. The main disadvantages stem from the potentially disruptive effects of bringing drug users together in a group. In most instances, drug users benefit more from the effects of normalizing their behaviour by seeing them during an ordinary surgery.

13

Working with other agencies

Berry Beaumont and Stefan Janikiewicz

As previous chapters have described, many drug users can be and are managed within general practice. Some drug users have complex and challenging needs. Counsellors and drug workers working in the surgery can provide help and support for these patients and their GP. Sometimes it is necessary to refer drug users to specialist services for aspects of their care, although the GP will retain responsibility for GMS. Such patients may later become stable enough to be transferred back to complete care in the practice.

Specialist service provision is patchy and inconsistent, with considerable variation from one district to another. There are around 475 specialist drug service providers in England, seeing about 84 000 clients at any one time.[1] About 50% of these are units within NHS trusts, the remainder being services provided by non-statutory organizations, mostly in the voluntary sector. Voluntary agencies receive much of their funding from NHS and local authority purchasers.

Community drug teams/street agencies

The first point of referral for the GP will usually be the local CDT or street agency. Community drug teams are health service agencies set up in the late 1980s in response to the HIV epidemic, to work collaboratively with GPs by providing counselling and other services to drug users, and supporting GPs in their prescribing role. Community drug teams exist in about half the health authorities in England, but their goal of increasing the involvement of GPs and other generic health professionals in the care of drug users has not been demonstrably achieved.[2] Street agencies are almost all non-statutory drop-in services, based in the community. In reality, there is considerable overlap between CDTs and street agencies, which between them provide a wide range of services.

Services provided by CDTs and street agencies

- Drop-in, information, advice

- Counselling – individual or group

- Needle exchange

- Safe sex advice and condom distribution

- Complementary therapies

- Outreach work

- Referral to residential detoxification and rehabilitation facilities

- Prescribing services (sometimes)

- Aftercare

Shared care

Shared care has become the central issue for policy makers and service providers, including GPs, who are struggling to meet demand for appropriate and effective treatment from an increasing number of drug users. It has been defined by the DoH as:[3]

The joint participation of specialists and GPs (and other agencies as appropriate) in the planned delivery of care for patients with a drug misuse problem, informed by an enhanced information exchange beyond routine discharge and referral letters. It may involve the day to day management by the GP of a patient's medical needs in relation to his or her drug misuse. Such arrangements would make explicit which clinician was responsible for different aspects of the patient's treatment and care. They may include prescribing substitute drugs in appropriate circumstances.

Shared care currently operates in many different ways, reflecting the heterogeneity of users' needs, GP skills and the extent and configuration of local drug services. In particular, the amount of support available from specialist services is very variable, and GPs are understandably anxious that shared care may in reality just mean they are left to deal with problems without adequate back-up.[4] Many shared-care arrangements could more appropriately be described as supported primary care. The GP shares the care of the drug user with a drugs worker based in the local community drug team or street agency. Most of these clients will be dependent opiate users on a methadone script. The drugs worker may run a regular clinic at the GP surgery and be responsible for most of the care, or the client may see him or her at the agency on a formal or informal basis, visiting the GP for the prescription and any other services the GP has agreed to provide. In these schemes, the GP is the only clinician and is in effect the specialist. Difficulties can arise if the client becomes too unstable or chaotic to be managed in general practice. The only option then is referral to the specialist NHS service where there may be long waiting lists.

Whatever the organizational arrangements for shared care, good communication and liaison between all those involved is vital to success. This includes other professionals involved, such as the community pharmacist who is dispensing. Areas of responsibility must be clearly defined. A comprehensive assessment of the drug user before deciding upon treatment (see Chapter 2) will help to identify the minority of clients for whom the lead clinician should be based in the specialist centre.

Specialist NHS drugs services

These are usually provided by a multi-disciplinary team directed by a consultant psychiatrist working in a DDU. Drug dependence units were established in the late 1960s and early 70s when the philosophy of working with drug users was that the problem lay in the substance being misused, specialist skills were necessary, and a relatively short detoxification with abstinence as the goal was the appropriate approach. This effectively deskilled generic health service professionals such as GPs, although in areas where DDUs were not set up, some GPs continued to treat drug-using patients. Because of the large increase in drug use in the 1980s, particularly in large cities, and the small number of DDUs, these services have been under tremendous pressure with long waits for users to be seen and accepted into treatment. This has been identified as one of the reasons why many referrals and first contacts do not lead to engagement in treatment.[5]

Since the advent of HIV and the development of a harm-minimization approach, and the recognition that substance misuse is just one component of a user's problems[6] there has been some shift in treatment policy in DDUs towards longer-term substitute prescribing and a recognition that general practice is an appropriate setting within which to care for drug-using patients. Recently, some new specialist units have been established, led by GPs. Their philosophy is more towards a keyworker-led strategy for patients, with all but the most chaotic users maintained in general practice.[7] Nevertheless, in many areas a tension still exists between the rigid approach of the DDU to scripting and associated expectations of client behaviour, and the treatment style of local GPs who may quite appropriately impose fewer conditions on users for whom they are prescribing on a long-term basis. Clinic regimens and the conditions attached to treatment were common reasons given by a sample of opiate users who had never sought help from a DDU.[8] This tension has contributed to the current situation in many areas of a mismatch between clients' needs and the services they are using. Chaotic and challenging users who 'fail' to keep to DDU rules find themselves being looked after in general practice, whilst some stable users on long-term scripts are taking up places on DDU programmes.

Is there an ideal model for shared care?

In some parts of the country, shared care is becoming established along the following lines. This may be a useful model for areas where services are at an earlier stage of development.

- Primary care and specialist services agree local protocols and procedures between them. These would include a common treatment philosophy, standardized assessment format and referral procedures. Clear criteria are established for which patients are seen in different parts of the service, and a number of workers in the specialist service are dedicated to working with, and supporting GPs and their patients.

- There may be a few local 'specialist' GPs who conduct assessment and interventions with minimal support from specialist services. These GPs work to agreed local standards, and participate in ongoing training and updating.

- Less experienced GPs accept drug users onto their lists, and agree to provide treatment within a formalized shared-care arrangement. The client is referred to the local drugs agency for an assessment, which may be done at the agency or in the surgery. The assessment is conducted in accordance with locally agreed protocols. A treatment plan and 'contract' is agreed which clarifies and apportions workload and responsibilities.

Checklist for dividing responsibilities within shared care

	Drugteam		GP
Initial drug history assessment	(✔)		( )
Initial urine screen	( )	either	( )
Check for IV sites	( )	either	( )
Annual weighing	( )	either	( )
Prescribing	( )		(✔)
Titration of methadone dose	( )	either	( )
Pharmacy liaison	( )		(✔)
Database notification	( )	either	( )
Counselling	(✔)	both	(✔)
Random urine testing – at least six-monthly	( )	either	( )
Hep B, Hep C and HIV testing and counselling	( )	either	( )
Hepatitis B immunization	( )	either	( )
Referral to secondary medical care	( )		(✔)
Sick certification	( )		(✔)
Housing letters	(✔)		( )
Legal reports	( )	either	( )
Probation liaison	(✔)		( )
Rehabilitation referral	(✔)		( )
Detoxification referral	(✔)		( )
Social services funding referral	(✔)		( )
Assistance with benefit problems	(✔)		( )
Child-protection issues	(✔)	both	(✔)

- Initial stabilization on a script can be undertaken by the agency, or by the GP. Stable clients are then prescribed for by the GP, with regular keyworker support. These workers can accompany clients to the surgery, conduct counselling and advice sessions at the practice, and/or participate in GP consultations if required.

- Drug users with more complex needs (mainly medical and psychiatric comorbidities) are managed by specialist services but registered with the GP for GMS. Specialist services offer additional support to GPs, and take back patients who have become unsuitable for GP management for whatever reason. In all instances there is both formal and informal joint working and regular communication with GPs.

- A locally established GP support and training scheme, led by one or more experienced GPs working as faciliators, co-ordinates the shared-care arrangements and organizes regular GP training and support forums. General practitioners who join the scheme will prescribe for and manage patients within locally agreed guidelines for which they receive payment. Payment may be conditional on GPs fulfilling certain criteria, including participation in training, and monitoring and auditing aspects of the care they provide. Participating GPs draw up their own list of 'gold standards' for care which might include the following:

  - hepatitis B status known and acted upon appropriately

  - urine screens before prescribing commences, and randomly twice-yearly thereafter

  - dispensing pharmacist identified and documented in notes

  - benzodiazepine prescribing limited to diazepam

  - goals reviewed with patient every six months.

For most districts, introducing this type of arrangement requires a review of the existing local service configuration, contracts and resourcing arrangements for primary and secondary care services. Progress towards the 'ideal' scenario will be incremental and relies on developing and maintaining good communication, understanding and trust between GPs and specialist services. Both these contributors to shared care need adequate resources to fulfil their roles effectively. Shifting the focus for the management of drug users into primary care must not result in an inappropriate reduction in specialist services.

Other health services

Crisis

Crisis may be associated with one or more of the following – acute intoxication, overdose, acute withdrawal; or physical, psychiatric or social comorbidities. Specialist crisis intervention services are rare, and the GP will need to liaise with accident and emergency departments, general medical and surgical services and the psychiatric service. GP 'out of hours' services may also be contacted by drug users, and GP co-operatives and commercial deputizing services should have a policy about how to respond appropriately to the kinds of problems that present at these times.

Psychiatric

Dual diagnosis is the term used to describe the status of drug users who have a concomitant mental health problem. There may be a causal, consequent or coincidental relationship between psychiatric morbidity and drug use. These patients are challenging to manage in psychiatric units, often because of behavioural problems. It may be difficult to get them admitted and for their drug use to be appropriately addressed during their stay in hospital. They have low rates of compliance with aftercare. There is considerable interest in the psychiatric and drug-addiction field in drawing up protocols for managements of these patients. Correct diagnosis can often only be achieved after in-patient observation in a psychiatric unit. A local psychiatrist with an interest in drug misuse is an essential requirement.

Patients with schizophrenic illness, manic depressive illness, or severe depression often have their illness exacerbated by drug misuse. Patients defined as having personality disorder are often not helped by in-patient psychiatric therapy. Drug misuse may be a major factor in their care management. A decision must be made whether a community psychiatric nurse or the drug worker is the relevant keyworker, with overall responsibility for care management in patients with dual diagnosis.

Specialist in-patient detoxification

In-patient drug misuse treatment services are available in a number of large cities. They provide medically supervised detoxification with counselling and support. The length of stay is usually four weeks. They may be particularly relevant for polydrug users with high levels of medical and psychiatric morbidity, although further research still needs to be done on their effectiveness compared with detoxification in other settings.[1]

Secondary care services for physical comorbidity and specialist obstetric care

Chapters 3 and 10, respectively, cover these aspects.

Services outside the NHS

Residential rehabilitation

Traditionally, these services have been provided by voluntary agencies or non-statutory agencies. There are 70 centres in the UK offering 1279 places.[9] Over half provide, or have access to detoxification facilities, and most offer programmes of between three and six months duration. Funding for a place is organized through the community care budget of the social services department of the user's local authority of residence. A local community drugs worker can usually organize the referral, and arrange for the necessary assessment and approval for funding. The availability of funding varies from place to place, and from year to year, and there may be long waits for admission.

Residential treatment programmes vary widely in concept and practice but fall broadly into four categories.[10]

1   *The concept house/therapeutic community* (Phoenix House is a well known example) – there is a strong reliance on the collective strength of peers and the value of intensive group work.

2 *The Christian rehabilitation house* – this may be strictly Christian (the resident must support the faith) or more loosely based on a Christian ethos that may motivate the staff but is not required of residents.

3 *Community integrated houses* – close links are formed with the local community and are seen as major elements of the rehabilitative process.

4 *12-step 'Minnesota model' houses* – these are based on the 12-step programme of Narcotics Anonymous, which subscribes to the disease model of addiction and relies heavily on self-help techniques. Narcotics Anonymous subsequently provides continued support beyond the residential phase.

Despite these differences in approach, residential centres share common features. Residents must be drug free and the centres provide a structured programme of psychological, educational and social therapy aimed at preparing the drug user to manage a drug-free life when back in society. Clients will usually have a feel for which type of rehabilitation will suit their needs. They may find it useful to have a copy of *The Rehabilitation Handbook*.[11]

Probation service

It has been estimated that about one fifth of people on probation are problem drug users,[12] although a recent study in London[13] suggested the proportion may be as high as a third. Treatment for drug misuse arranged during a period of supervision by the probation service rarely forms part of the formal sentence of the court – only 3% of probation orders made in 1993 had an additional requirement for drug treatment. Probation services are now required to have a drugs policy and strategy. When treating a drug user in general practice, it is useful to ask if he or she has a probation officer, and to make contact by telephone. Probation officers often see these clients on a regular basis. It is helpful to them to know what treatment strategy the GP is following, and they can provide useful feedback to the GP with their perceptions of how the user is coping.

Police

It is appropriate for GPs to be aware that most police forces operate some form of arrest referral scheme, intended to exploit the opportunity provided by arrest to encourage drug users to seek treatment. The schemes vary from simply offering contact telephone numbers for drug treatment services, to providing a more structured response with drug workers on site or on call. *The Task Force Report*[1] has recommended that arrest referral schemes be provided at every police station. Police surgeons, many of whom are also GPs, are involved in assessment and treatment of drug users in police custody. They should also take the opportunity to put drug users in contact with appropriate treatment services, which can best be provided or co-ordinated by their GP.

Complementary therapies

Therapies such as hypnotherapy, shiatsu and acupuncture may be offered by drugs agencies as an adjunct or alternative to more conventional treatments. There is a scarcity of research data to support claims of effectiveness, but these therapies are popular with clients and they do apparently attract some drug users, e.g. cocaine users, into treatment services.[14]

Self-help networks

In its broadest sense, self-help refers to the support that drug users and their families and friends can draw on outside of formal drug treatment. Effective support contributes to the success of users in achieving whatever goals they have set for themselves. There is no national self-help organization of drug users in England, unlike other countries such as Holland and Australia, but a number of groups exist at local level.

Narcotics Anonymous (NA) has 350 groups in England, and follows the 12-step approach used by Alcoholics Anonymous. Reference to God appears in six of the 12 steps, which some clients may not find an acceptable ethos, although NA is not run by any particular religious set. Families Anonymous uses a similar approach to help family members to resist colluding with a drug misuser.

ADFAM National provides a range of services to support families, including a telephone helpline and training for family support groups. A recent survey of treatment agencies[15] has shown that the support offered by them to families is usually limited to telephone advice and information leaflets. Few provide counselling or family support groups. General practitioners are in a good position to counsel family members whom they may already know well if they have been registered with them for some time.

There are a great number of positive anecdotes about the usefulness of self-help networks and GPs should be able to give users information about how to access them.

Other services

GPs may also need to liaise with a number of other services:

- housing departments
- welfare benefits advice
- education service
- young people's projects.

Development of services

Following the publication of the White Paper *Tackling Drugs Together*[16] local responsibility for developing and implementing a strategy for tackling problem drug misuse in England has recently been passed to the newly established Drug Action Teams (DATs). These now operate in every district and have multi-agency representation at executive level. General practitioners are not often directly involved. However, GPs may be represented on the associated drug reference groups (DRGs) that have broad membership and have been set up to advise the DATs. Responsibility for commissioning services still rests with health authority and local authority purchasers, and it is in this arena that GPs can be most influential. GP involvement in commissioning varies from district to district. GPs may be fundholders, purchasing services for the practice population directly, or involved in purchasing and commissioning for localities or districts through membership of local GP organizations working in conjunction with the health authority. In order to develop services appropriate to a primary care-led service for drug users, as for any other patient group, GPs must ensure that the needs of these patients are clearly articulated and provided for. The provision of appropriate training and resources to support GPs in their provider role must also be addressed.

Appendix – useful contacts

ADFAM National: Waterbridge House, 32–36 Loman Street, London, SE1 0EE, Tel: 0171 928 8900
Information, advice, counselling. National helpline for families and friends of users.

Families Anonymous: The Doddington and Rollo Community Association, Charlotte Despard Avenue, London, SW11 5JE, Tel: 0171 498 4680
Advice and support groups for families and friends.

ISDD (Institute for the Study of Drug Dependence): Waterbridge House, 32–36 Loman Street, London, SE1 0EE, Tel: 0171 928 1211
Comprehensive library service and research department. Many publications including very informative bi-monthly magazine called *Drug Link*.

NA (Narcotics Anonymous): UK Service Office, PO Box 1980, London, N19 3LS, Tel: 0171 351 6794 (Helpline) and 0171 351 6066 (Recorded meeting list)
Self-help fellowship. Groups located throughout UK.

National drugs helpline: Tel: 0800 77 66 00 – 24 hours
Free information and advice and support about drug issues.

Release: 388 Old Street, London, EC1V 9LT, Tel: 0171 729 9904, 24 hour emergency help-line: 0171 603 8654
Telephone advice for legal emergencies, and drug information and advice.

SCODA (Standing Conference on Drug Abuse): Waterbridge House, 32–36 Loman Street, London, SE1 0EE, Tel: 0171 928 9500
National co-ordinating and representative body for drug services and those working with drug users. Dial-and-listen service for details of drug agencies. Dial 100 and ask for Freephone Drug Problems.

Acknowledgement

Thanks are due to the Substance Misuse Management Project of Brent and Harrow Health Authority for helpful suggestions based on their work with local GPs developing a model for shared care.

14

Drugs and the law

Greg Poulter

There is nothing simple or straightforward about drug legislation presently in force in England and Wales. It is complex and involved and to the uninitiated can appear to be an impenetrable barrier. The laws in relation to the unlawful use of 'street' drugs are also very severe and the consequences of transgressing the law are dire, involving loss of good character and, frequently, liberty. The number of individuals coming into contact with the Criminal Justice System in relation to drugs is rising each year and is approaching 100 000, of whom the significant majority are young people.

The aim of various pieces of legislation is, on the one hand, to limit misuse and availability of various drugs that are considered to be harmful to individuals and society as a whole, and on the other to allow sufficient flexibility for the legitimate therapeutic use of some of these drugs.

There are two major statutes that regulate this area: The Medicines Act 1968 (MA) and The Misuse of Drugs Act 1971 (MDA) with its associated Misuse of Drugs Regulations (MDRegs).

The Medicines Act

This Act deals with medicinal products. These are any substances or articles that are manufactured, sold or supplied, wholly or mainly to be administered for a medicinal purpose, or which are ingredients of something that is to be administered for a medicinal purpose.

The inspiration for the MA was the protection of the public from defective or flawed medicines in that the Act regulates the production and supply of medicinal products. It is not a piece of legislation that is primarily aimed at combating the illegal possession, or supply of 'street' drugs.

The MA creates three groups of medicinal products:

1   The general sale list

2   Pharmacy medicines

3   Prescription-only medicines (POMs).

The general sale list

A list of medicinal products over which there is the least control of the three categories and which do not need to be sold under the supervision of a pharmacist.

Pharmacy medicines

All the medicines that are not in the other two lists are automatically placed in this category. These medicines can only be sold under the supervision of a pharmacist.

Prescription-only medicine

Prescription-only medicines can only be supplied under a prescription and are viewed as only suitable to be supplied under the supervision of a doctor. Injectable medicinal products are POMs, including ampoules of sterile water.

The Misuse of Drugs Act

This Act seeks to regulate the importation and exportation, production and possession of certain drugs that are considered 'dangerous or otherwise harmful'. Such drugs are called controlled drugs. The Act provides delegated powers to make regulations, known as the Misuse of Drugs Regulations.

The MDA creates a number of criminal offences making it an offence to possess controlled drugs. Thus section 5(1) states:

... it shall not be lawful for a person to have a controlled drug in their possession.

Section 4(1) makes it an offence:

to supply or offer to supply a controlled drug to another.

Section 5(3) makes it an offence:

for a person to have a controlled drug in their possession, whether lawfully or not, with intent to supply it to another.

If this was where the law stopped then GPs and pharmacists could not undertake their work, as every time they provided their patient with dihydrocodeine or temazepam they would be committing an offence. Fortunately, the law provides a number of exceptions to the above offences enabling the GP to prescribe and supply appropriate drugs.

What is a 'controlled drug'?

The MDA does not attempt to provide a definition of the dangerous drugs that it seeks to regulate. Rather it sets out a series of lists of drugs that are described as controlled drugs. There are two groups of lists, the Classes and the Schedules.

Classes

The first group is found in Schedule 2 to the MDA and is referred to as the Classes. As might be expected, controlled drugs are not all treated the same under the law. There is a type of hierarchy of danger, and those drugs which are viewed as the most dangerous and harmful and therefore attract the greatest penalty are placed in *Class A*. Diamorphine, desomorphine, cocaine and lysergide are examples of drugs found in Class A and the maximum penalty for unlawfully supplying one of these groups is life imprisonment and/or an unlimited fine.

In *Class B* are drugs viewed as less serious, such as amphetamine, methylamphetamine, cannabis and codeine. The maximum penalty for unlawfully supplying a drug in this class is 14 years and/or an unlimited fine.

Class C contains the remaining controlled drugs, such as bromazepam, diazepam and temazepam, for which the maximum penalty for supplying is five years and/or an unlimited fine.

In many cases any substance that is structurally derived from, or is in any stereoisometric form of, or salt of, the substance named in the class, is also controlled.

The sole function of the Classes is to set out the level of penalty for an offence associated with a controlled drug.

Schedules

The second group of lists is found in five Schedules contained in the Misuse of Drug Regulations 1985 (as amended). The Schedules deal with far more complex areas of law than the Classes. The Schedule in which a particular controlled drug is placed dictates who can lawfully possess or supply it, how it must be stored, whether a GP can prescribe it, the form of the prescription, etc.

Drugs in Schedule 1 are viewed as possessing no therapeutic value, so they cannot be prescribed. In this schedule are lysergide and (for some, controversially) cannabis. The remaining four Schedules impose different levels of control on the drugs contained within them. Those in Schedule 2 are subject to the most control, with Schedule 5 the least. Schedule 2 drugs include dihydrocodeine, cocaine, diamorphine, methadone, pethidine. Schedule 3 drugs include chlorophentermine, mazindol and temazepam. Schedule 4 includes bromazepam, diazepam, lorazepam and nitrazepam.

Section 5 of the MDA makes it an offence to possess a controlled drug. However, under Regulation 10(1) of the Misuse of Drug Regulations a GP or pharmacist may possess and supply a drug contained in Schedules 2 to 4. It is this regulation which gives authority to GPs to have a controlled drug in their possession and to administer it according to their clinical judgement. However, a specific licence is required before GPs can prescribe cocaine, diamorphine and dipipanone to treat dependency on these drugs, although any doctor can prescribe these drugs for other purposes. Any doctor may prescribe methadone for an addict.

As far as the patient is concerned, Regulation 10(2) protects them as follows:

a person may have in his possession any drug specified in Schedules 2 or 3 for administration for medical, dental or veterinary purposes in accordance with the direction of a practitioner.

As a general rule, controlled drugs contained in Schedules 2 to 4 can only be supplied by a GP or pharmacist, and those in Schedules 2 and 3 can only be lawfully possessed by members of the public if these drugs have been *prescribed* to them. Anyone can possess a

Schedule 4 drug provided it is a medicinal product, i.e. in the form in which it is intended to be taken for medicinal purposes.

There are of course other categories of people who might possess or supply a controlled drug without committing an offence, providing they are doing so in the course of their profession or business, for example police officers, those engaged in the business of the post office or forensic examination in a laboratory, couriers, etc.

Any person may possess Schedule 5 drugs. These are various dilute, small-dose, non-injectable products that can often be sold without prescription by a pharmacist. They include cough medicines, anti-diarrhoea agents and mild painkillers.

Once brought, Schedule 5 drugs cannot be supplied to someone else, an injunction that is rarely enforced.

Each controlled drug has two listings; one in the Classes and one in the Schedules. For example, diamorphine is in Class A and Schedule 2, and cannabis is in Class B and Schedule 1.

The Act allows considerable flexibility to the Home Office to amend the Schedules and Classes. It is a relatively simple matter for new substances to be brought into control, as with anabolic steroids that were recently introduced into the system into Class C Schedule 4. Existing controlled drugs can also be moved within the Schedules as with temazepam which, although it remains in Class C, was moved from Schedule 4 to Schedule 3. Thus it is now an offence to possess temazepam unless personally prescribed for, whereas formerly it was only an offence to supply it other than under a prescription. There is a procedure that must be undertaken by the Home Office before such amendments can be made. This includes wide consultation, particularly with the Advisory Committee on the Misuse of Drugs.

Double-scripting

If a patient obtains a prescription of controlled drugs from Dr A, and then obtains a second prescription from Dr B without disclosing the first prescription, the patient will be in lawful possession of the controlled drugs from Dr A, but in unlawful possession of the drugs from Dr B.

Dishonestly obtaining controlled drugs

The Misuse of Drugs Regulation 10(2) provides that if patients make a declaration or statement to a prescribing doctor that 'was false in any (material) particular, for the purpose of obtaining the supply or prescription', they will be in unlawful possession of those prescribed drugs. Consequently, if a patient misleads a GP about the need for a particular drug, for example a patient lies about being dependent on heroin so as to obtain a methadone 'script', he or she is in unlawful possession of the methadone even though it has been prescribed to him or her by a GP.

Common offences

It is helpful for professionals who are working with individuals who are using 'street' drugs to have a basic understanding of the more common offences.

The majority of people who come into contact with the Criminal Justice System are arrested for simple *possession* of a controlled drug. For the prosecution to establish this offence it is necessary to show:

1   that the substance was in the possession or control of the defendant

2   that the substance was in fact a controlled drug

3   that the defendant knew of the existence of the substance.

Many people arrested by police in possession of a small quantity of a controlled drug will not be charged but will receive a 'caution'; that is a formal warning. Even if they are charged with the offence of possession and have to attend the court the most likely sentence is a fine. It is unusual for an individual to receive a prison sentence for simple possession.

With regards to *supply* offences, there are a number of different offences. The two main ones are possession with intent to supply, and actual supply. A wide range of activities involving controlled drugs can be classified as supplying and thus incur the possibility of a serious sentence. It is not necessary to show some benefit accruing to suppliers to make them guilty of the crime. If an individual simply gives or shares a controlled drug with another he or she commits the offence, so sharing a 'spliff/joint' with a friend would be supplying cannabis. It would be an offence of 'possession with intent to supply' for a person to look after an Ecstasy tablet for a friend. If two people club together to buy some cannabis, the person who goes to buy the drug would be committing a similar offence.

The consequences, on conviction, for the most minor of supply-type offences are frequently very serious. The 'entry point' for sentence is normally custodial. The supply of Class A drugs, even social supply of small amounts, for no profit, will commonly attract a prison sentence of between 18 months and three years. Where there appears to be a profit motive, then three- to five-year sentences are very frequent. The fact that the defendant has no previous convictions does not substantially affect the sentence.

The cost of 'street' drugs to the user is a good indicator of availability. Shortages should push the prices up while gluts can cause the price to fall. However it is a remarkable, if not disturbing, feature of the 'street scene' that prices are actually very stable, with little variation over considerable periods of time. LSD 'tabs' sell at about £3 each, amphetamine at around £10 per gram and Ecstasy at £8 per tablet. Heroin and cocaine can cost as little as £40 per gram. These drugs are also readily available in most parts of the UK.

The importance of GPs working in co-operation with local drug projects to deal effectively with drug dependency issues cannot be over emphasized. Many of these local agencies are able to provide guidance and support to GPs and their drug-dependent patients and they will provide assessments and make recommendations for prescribing. However GPs cannot delegate their clinical decisions to others. It is the GP's legal responsibility to ensure that the appropriate prescription is made.

Drugs and driving

There is an offence of driving a motor vehicle while unfit through drink or drugs. Most successful drink-driving convictions are based on the legal presumption that if the proportion of alcohol to breath is over a certain level then the driver is unfit and the offence is committed. No such provision is available for drug-driving matters. In these cases the prosecution must prove:

1   that the driver was unfit, often based on the evidence of the medical examiner called by the police

2   that the driver was unfit through drugs.

The law relating to driving while unfit applies equally to prescribed and non-prescribed drugs. It is not a defence to a charge of driving while unfit through drugs that the driver was unfit through a prescribed drug, that had been taken in accordance with the GP's directions.

There is grave concern on the part of many senior police officers that there are significant numbers of drivers who are unfit through drugs and who are not identified. The concern is such that a major piece of research is presently under way to assess the extent of the problem and there are calls for a radical overhaul of the law (Association of Chief Police Officers Conference, 1996).

Prescribing GPs do have responsibilities in this area. Guidelines are issued by the Driver and Vehicle Licensing Authority (DVLA) with regard to driving and drugs and these are easily obtainable from either HMSO or the DVLA. It is possible that a prescribing GP could be viewed as negligent if he or she does not advise a patient as to the dangers of driving if the medication prescribed might affect driving ability. With regard to prescribed methadone, the DVLA considers that a person should not be driving if he or she is in receipt of injectable methadone. If patients receive the drug in any other form then it is up to the GP's clinical judgement as to whether they should continue to drive.

References and further reading

Chapter 1

1   UK Department of Health and Social Security, Medical Working Group on Drug Dependence (1984) *Guidelines on Good Clinical Practice in the Treatment of Drug Misuse.* DHSS, London.

2   White Paper (1994) *Tackling Drugs Together: A Strategy for England 1995–1998.* HMSO, London.

3   Welsh Office (1995) *Forward Together. A Strategy to Combat Drug and Alcohol Misuse in Wales.* Welsh Office.

4   Report of the Ministerial Drugs Task Force (1994) *Drugs in Scotland: Meeting the Challenge.* Home and Health Department, Scottish Office.

5   Report of an Independent Review of Drug Treatment Services in England (1996) *The Task Force to Review Services for Drug Misusers.* Department of Health, London.

6   Report of the Departmental Committee on Morphine and Heroin Addiction (1926) HMSO, London.

7   Spear B (1994) The early Years of the 'British System' in Practice. In *Heroin Addiction and Drug Policy. The British System* (eds J Strang and M Gossop). Oxford University Press, Oxford. pp. 3–28.

8   Report (1961) *UK Interdepartmental Committee on Drug Addiction.* (Chaired by Sir Russell Brain). HMSO, London.

9   Second Report (1965) *UK Interdepartmental Committee on Drug Addiction.* (Chaired by Sir Russell Brain). HMSO, London.

10   UK Department of Health and Social Security (1982) *Treatment and Rehabilitation: Report of the Advisory Council on the Misuse of Drugs (ACMD): Central Funding Initiative.* HMSO, London.

11   Glanz A and Taylor C (1986) Findings of a national survey of the role of general practitioners in the treatment of opiate misuse (3 parts). *BMJ.* **294**: 427–30.

12   Report by the Advisory Council on the Misuse of Drugs (1988) *AIDS and Drug Misuse Part 1.* HMSO, London.

13   Stimson, GV (1996) Has the United Kingdom averted an epidemic of HIV-1 infection among drug injectors? *Addiction.* **91**(8): 1085–8.

14   Stimson GV, Hunter GM, Donoghoe MC *et al.* (1996) HIV prevalence in community-wide samples of injecting drug users in London (1990–1993). *AIDS.* **10**: 657–66.

15   Unlinked Anonymous HIV Surveys Steering Group (1995) *Unlinked Anonymous HIV Prevention Monitoring Programme: England and Wales.* Department of Health, London.

16   Haw S, Frischer M, Donoghoe MC *et al.* (1992) The importance of multisite sampling in determining the prevalence of HIV among drug injectors in Glasgow and London. *AIDS.* **6**: 517–18.

17   Peters AD, Reid M and Griffin SG (1994) Edinburgh drug users: are they injecting and sharing less? *AIDS.* **8**: 521–8.

18   Waller T and Holmes R (1995) Hepatitis C: scale and impact in Britain. *Drug Link.* September/October, 8–11. ISDD, London.

19   BMA Report on Drug Misuse (1997) (*in press*).

20   Leitner M, Shapland J and Wiles P (1993) *Drug Usage and Drugs Prevention: the views and habits of the general public.* HMSO, London.

21   Parker H, Measham F and Aldridge J (1995) Drug futures: changing patterns of drug use among English youth. *Research Monograph. 7.* ISDD, London.

22   Mott J and Mirlees-Black C (1995) *Self-Reported Drug Misuse in England and Wales: findings from the 1992 British Crime Survey.* Home Office, London.

23   Balding J (1995) *Young People in 1994.* University of Exeter, Exeter.

24   Frischer M (1992) Estimated Prevalence of Injecting Drug Use in Glasgow. *British Journal of Addiction.* **37**: 235–44.

25   Scott R, Gruer L, Wilson P *et al.* (1995) Glasgow has an innovative scheme for encouraging GPs to manage drug misusers. Letter. *BMJ.* **310**: 464–5.

26   The Royal College of General Practitioners (1995) *Managing Drug Users in General Practice. Why? How?* Report of a conference organised by the HIV/AIDS working party, RCGP, London.

27   General Medical Services Committee (1996) *Core Services: Taking the Initiative.* British Medical Association, London.

Chapter 2

1   Stimson GV, Hayden D, Hunter G *et al.* (1995) *Drug Users' Help-Seeking and Views of Services.* A Report prepared for the Task Force to review Services for Drug Misusers.

2   Resource and Service Development Centre (1996) *Shared Care, Shared Barriers. Reviewing Shared-Care Arrangements for Drug Misusers.* RSDC, Leeds.

3   Bury J (1995) Supporting GPs in Lothian to care for drug users. *International Journal of Drug Policy.* **6**(4): 267–73.

Chapter 3

1   Home Office (1995) Statistics of drug addicts notified to the Home Office. United Kingdom (1994) *Home Office Statistical Bulletin.* 19 July, Home Office, London.

2   Report by the Advisory Council on the Misuse of Drugs (1993) *AIDS and Drug Misuse Update.* HMSO, London.

3   Hindler C, Nazareth I, King M *et al.* (1995) Drug users' views on general practitioners. *BMJ.* **310**: 300.

4   Leaver EJ, Elford J, Morris JK *et al.* (1992) Use of general practice by intravenous heroin users on a methadone programme. *British Journal of General Practice.* **42**: 465–8.

5   Ronald PJM, Witcomb JC, Robertson JR *et al.* (1992) Problems of drug abuse, HIV and AIDS: The burden of care in one general practice. *British Journal of General Practice.* **42**: 232–5.

6   Rhodes T, Donoghue M, Hunter G *et al.* (1994) Sexual behaviour of drug injectors in London: implications for HIV transmission and HIV prevention. *Addiction.* **89**(9): 1085–95.

7   Cohen J (1994) Problem drug users: a problem for the GP? *Practitioner.* **238**: 715–18.

8   Gerada C, Orgel M and Strang J (1992) Health Clinics for Problem Drug Users. *Health Trends.* **24**: 68–9.

9   Telfer I and Clulow C (1990) Heroin misusers: what they think of their general practitioners. *British Journal of Addiction.* **85**: 137–40.

10   Zamora-Quezada JC, Dinerman H, Stadecker MJ *et al.* (1988) Muscle and skin infarction after free-basing cocaine (crack). *Annals Internal Medicine.* **108**: 564–6.

11   Murphy M, Pomeroy L, Tynan M *et al.* Cervical cytological screening in HIV-infected women in Dublin – a six-year review. *International Journal of Sexually Transmitted Diseases – AIDS.* **6**(4): 262–6.

12   Guillebaud J (1994) Contraception – your questions answered (2nd edn). Churchill Livingstone, London.

13   Datt N and Feinmann C (1990) Providing health care for drug users? *British Journal of Addiction.* **85**: 1571–5.

14   Smith HM, Alexander GJ, Webb G *et al.* (1992) Hepatitis B and delta virus infection among 'at risk' populations in south east London. *Journal of Epidemiology and Community Health.* **46**: 144–7.

15   Wong V, Wreghitt TG, Alexander GJM (1996) Prospective study of hepatitis B vaccination in patients with chronic hepatitis C. *BMJ.* **312**: 1336–7.

16   Farrell M, Battersby M and Strang J (1990) Screening for hepatitis B and vaccinating of injecting drug users in NHS drug treatment services. *British Journal of Addiction.* **85**: 1657–9.

17   Rumi M, Colombo M, Romeo R *et al.* (1991) Suboptimal response to hepatitis B vaccine in drug users. *Archives Internal Medicine.* **151**: 574–8.

18   Mattson L, Weiland O and Glaumman H (1995) Long term follow up of chronic post-transfusion non-A, non-B hepatitis: clinical and histological outcome. *Liver.* **3**: 184–8.

19   Department of Health (1995) Unlinked anonymous HIV prevalence monitoring programme: England and Wales: Data to end of 1993. (Chair Dr E Rubery) Report from the unlinked anonymous HIV surveys steering group, Department of Health, London.

20   Birthistle K, Maguire H, Atkinson P *et al.* Who's having HIV tests? An audit of HIV test requests in an large London teaching hospital. *Health Trends.* **28**(2): 60–3.

Chapter 4

1   Prochaska JO and Di Clemente CC (1982) Towards a comprehensive model of change. In *Treating Addictive Behaviours: processes of change* (WR Miller and N Heather eds). Plenum Press, New York. pp. 3–27.

2   Sanchez-Craig M and Wilkinson DA (1987) Brief treatments for alcohol and drug problems: Practical and methodological issues. In *Addictive Behaviour: prevention and early intervention* (T Loberg, W Miller, PE Nathan and GA Marlatt eds). Swets & Zeitlinger, Amsterdam. pp. 233–52.

3   Miller WR (1989) Increasing motivation for change. In *Handbook of Alcoholism Treatment Approaches: effective alternatives* (RK Hester and WR Miller eds). Pergamon Press, New York. pp. 67–80.

Further reading

Miller W and Rollnick S (eds) (1991) *Motivational Interviewing.* Guildford Press, Guildford.

Mulleady G (ed.) (1992) *Counselling Drug Users about HIV and AIDS.* Blackwell Scientific Publications, Oxford.

Chapter 5

1   Edwards G (1971) *Unreason in an Age of Reason*. Royal Society of Medicine, London.

2   Hart G (1996) *Drug Cultures in Context*. MRC News. Medical Research Council, London.

3   Marlatt AG and Tapert SF (1993) Harm reduction: reducing the risk of addictive behaviours. In *Addictive Behaviours Across the Life Span* (J Baer, AG Marlatt and J McMahon eds). Sage Publications, London.

4   Department of Health and Social Security (1984) *Guidelines for Good Clinical Practice in the Treatment of Drug Misuse*. DHSS, London.

5   Department of Health, Scottish Home and Health Department, Welsh Office (1991) *Drug Misuse and Dependence: Guidelines on Clinical Management*. HMSO, London.

6   Parker H, Measham F and Aldridge J (1995) Drug futures: changing patterns of drug use among English youth. *Research Monograph*. **7**. ISDD, London.

7   Donovan J and Jesser R (1985) Structure of problem behaviour in adolescence and young adulthood. *Journal of Consulting and Clinical Psychology*. **53**: 890–904.

8   Pandina RJ and Schuele JA (1983) Psychosocial correlates of alcohol and drug use of adolescent students and adolescents in treatment. *Journal of Studies in Alcohol*. **44**: 950–73.

9   Barrett MJ and Trepper TS (1991) Treating Women Drug Abusers who were Victims of Childhood Sex Abuse. In *Feminism and Addiction*. Haworth Press, New York.

10   Institute for the Study of Drug Dependence (1997) *Drug Misuse in Britain 1996*. ISDD, London.

11   Department of Health Statistical Bulletin (1996) *Drug Misuse Statistics 1996/24*. December 1996. Department of Health, London.

12   Welsh I (1993) *Trainspotting*. Martin Secker & Warburg, London.

13   Inchiardi JA (1979) Heroin use and street crime. *Crime and delinquency*. **25**: 325–46.

14   d'Urso P and Hobbs R (1989) Aggression and the general practitioner. *BMJ*. **298**: 97–8.

15   Greenwood J (1992) Unpopular patients: GPs' attitudes to drug users. *Drug Link*. July/August, 8–10. ISDD, London.

16   Wilson P, Watson R and Ralston GE (1995) Supporting problem drug users: improving methadone maintenance in general practice. *British Journal of General Practice*. **45**: 454–5.

17   Martin E (1987) Managing drug addiction – the reality behind the guidelines. *Journal of Royal Society of Medicine*. **80**: 305–7.

18   King MB (1989) Psychological and social problems in HIV infection: interviews with general practitioners in London. *BMJ*. **299**: 713–17.

19   Gronbladh L, Ohlund LS and Gunne LM (1990) Mortality in heroin addiction, impact of methadone treatment. *Acta Psychiatrics Scandinavia*. **82**: 223–7.

20   Bennet T and Wright R (1986) Opioid users' attitudes towards and use of NHS clinics, general practitioners and private doctors. *British Journal of Addiction*. **81**: 757–63.

21   Martin E. Unpublished statistics of ten years' caring for drug users in one practice in Bedfordshire 1985–95.

Chapter 6

1   Farrell M, Ward J, Mattick R *et al*. (1994) Methadone maintenance treatment in opiate dependence: a review. *BMJ*. **309**: 997–1001.

2   Ward J, Mattick R and Hall W (1992) *Key Issues in Methadone Maintenance Treatment*. New South Wales University Press, Kensington, New South Wales.

3   Sorensen JL (1996) Methadone treatment for opiate addicts. *BMJ*. **313**: 245–6.

4   McKeganey NP and Boddy FA (1988) General practitioners and opiate-abusing patients. *Journal of the Royal College of General Practitioners*. **38**: 73–5.

5   Wilson P, Watson R and Ralston GE (1995) Supporting problem drug users: improving methadone maintenance in general practice. *British Journal of General Practice.* **45**: 454–5.

6   Greenwood J (1990) Creating a new drug service in Edinburgh. *BMJ.* **300**: 587–9.

7   Wilson P, Watson R and Ralston GE (1994) Methadone maintenance in general practice: patients, workload, and outcomes. *BMJ.* **309**: 641–4.

8   Greenwood J (1996) Shared care with general practitioners for Edinburgh's drug users. *International Journal of Drug Policy.* **7**(1): 19–22.

9   Preston A (1996) *The Methadone Briefing.* Martindale Pharmaceuticals, London. (Distributed by ISDD, Waterbridge House, 32–36, Loman Street, London, SE1 0EE.)

10   Scott RTA, Burnett SJ and McNulty H (1994) Supervised administration of methadone by pharmacists (letter). *BMJ.* **308**: 1438.

11   Strang J, Sheridan J and Barber N (1996) Prescribing injectable and oral methadone to opiate addicts: results from the 1995 national postal survey of community pharmacists in England and Wales. *BMJ.* **313**: 270–2.

Chapter 7

1   Department of Health (1996) *Drug Misuse Statistics 1995.* Department of Health, London.

2   Strang J, Johns A and Caan W (1993) Cocaine in the UK – 1991. *British Journal of Psychiatry.* **162**: 1–13.

3   Home Office (1996) *Statistics of Drug Addicts Notified to the Home Office UK 1995.* Home Office, London.

4   Seivewright N and McMahon C (1996) Misuse of amphetamines and related drugs. *Advances in Psychiatric Treatment.* **2**: 211–18.

5   Fleming PM and Roberts D (1994) Is the prescription of amphetamine justified as a harm reduction measure? *Journal of Royal Society of Health.* June, 127–31.

6   The Centre for Research on Drugs and Health Behaviour (1993) Ecstasy and the rave scene: new drug, new subculture, old problems? *Executive Summary.* No. 25.

7   McGuire PK, Cope H and Fahy T (1994) Diversity of psychopathology associated with use of 3,4-methylenedioxmethamphetamine ('Ecstasy'). *British Journal of Psychiatry.* **165**: 391–5.

Further reading

Bock GR and Whelan J (eds) (1992) Cocaine: scientific and social dimensions. *Ciba Foundation Symposium 166.* John Wiley & Sons, Chichester.

Ghodse H (1995) *Drugs and Addictive Behaviour, a Guide to Treatment* (2nd edn). Blackwell Science, Oxford.

Tyler A (1995) *Street Drugs.* Hodder & Stoughton, London.

Chapter 8

1   Darke S (1995) The use of benzodiazepines amongst injecting drug users. *Drug and Alcohol Review.* **13**: 63–9.

2   Simpson R (1993) Benzodiazepines in general practice. In *Benzodiazepine dependence* (ed. C. Hallstrom). Oxford University Press, Oxford. pp. 252–66.

3   Committee for the Review of Medicines (1980) Systematic review of the benzodiazepines: guidelines for data sheets. *BMJ.* **80**: 910–11.

4   Royal College of Psychiatrists (1988) Benzodiazepines and dependence. 'A College Statement'. *Bulletin of the Royal College of Psychiatrists.* **12**: 107–8.

5   Catalan J and Gath DH (1985) Benzodiazepines in general practice: a time for a decision. *BMJ.* **290**: 1374–6.

6   Seivewright N, Donmall M and Daly C (1993) Benzodiazepines in the illicit drugs scene: the UK picture and some dilemmas. *The International Journal of Drug Policy.* **4**(1): 42–8.

7　　Parker H, Measham F and Aldridge J (1995) Drug futures: changing patterns of drug use among English youth. *Research Monograph.* **7**. ISDD, London.

8　　Strang J, Griffiths P, Abbey J *et al.* (1994) Survey of use of injected benzodiazepines amongst drug users in Britain. *BMJ.* **308**: 1082.

9　　Seivewright N and Dougal W (1993) Withdrawal symptoms from high dose benzodiazepines in poly drug users. *Drug and Alcohol Dependence.* **32**: 15–23.

10　　Ashton H (1984) Benzodiazepine withdrawal: an unfinished story. *BMJ.* **288**: 1135–40.

11　　Ashton H (1994) The treatment of benzodiazepine dependence. *Addiction.* **89**: 1535–41.

12　　King M, Gabe J, Williams P *et al.* (1990) Long-term use of benzo-diazepines: the views of patients. *British Journal of General Practice.* **40**: 194–6.

Chapter 9

1　　Strang J, Darke S, Hall W *et al.* (1996) Heroin Overdose; the case for take-home naloxone. *British Medical Journal.* **312**: 1435.

Chapter 10

1　　Home Office Statistical Bulletin (1995) *Statistics of Drug Addicts Notified to the Home Office, United Kingdom, 1994.* Issue 17/95. HMSO, London.

2　　Department of Health Statistical Bulletin (1996) *Drug Misuse Statistics Bulletin.* 1996/24. Department of Health, London.

3　　Condie RG, Brown SS, Akter MI *et al.* (1989) Acute urinary screening for drugs of addiction ... usefulness of side room testing. *British Journal of Addiction.* **84**: 1543–5.

4   The second report of the National Local Authority Forum on Drugs Misuse in conjunction with the Standing Conference on Drug Abuse (1989) *Issues for Policy Makers: drug using parents and their children.* September 1989.

5   Hepburn M (1993) Drug misuse in pregnancy. *Current Obstetrics and Gynaecology.* **3**: 54–8.

6   Gerada C (1995) Pregnancy and drug abuse: complications and management issues. *European Addiction Research.* **1**: 146–50.

7   Hepburn M (1993) Drug use in pregnancy. *British Journal of Hospital Medicine.* **49**(1): 51–5.

8   Siney C, Kidd M, Walkinshaw S *et al.* (1995) Opiate dependency in pregnancy. *British Journal of Midwifery.* **3**(2): 69–73.

9   Boag F (1991) Hepatitis B – heterosexual transmission and vaccination strategies. *International Journal of STD and AIDS.* **2**: 318–24.

10   Waller T and Holmes R (1995) Hepatitis C: scale and impact in Britain. *Drug Link.* September/October, 8–11. ISDD, London.

11   MacCullum R, France R and Jones M (1988) The effects of pregnancy on the progression of HIV. *Abstract 4032.* IVth International Conference on AIDS, Stockholm.

12   Taylor A (1997) Study on drug using women, Glasgow, 1991/2. Personal communication.

13   Van Baar A (1991) The Development of Infants of Drug Dependent Mothers. Swets & Zeitlinger, Amsterdam.

Chapter 11

1   Williams T, Wetton N and Moon A (1989) *Health for Life 1 and 2.* Nelson, London.

2   Balding J (1995) *Young People in 1994: the health-related behaviour questionnaire results.* Schools Health Education Unit, Exeter University.

3   Goddard E (1996) *Teenage Drinking in 1994.* HMSO, London.

4   Diamond A (1995) *Smoking Amongst Secondary School Children in 1994.* HMSO, London.

5   Balding J (1994) *Young People and Illegal Drugs, 1989–1995 – Facts and Predictions.* Schools Health Education Unit, Exeter University.

6   Institute for the Study of Drug Dependence (1997) *Drug Misuse in Britain 1996.* ISDD, London.

7   Institute for the Study of Drug Dependence (1993) *National Audit of Drug Misuse in Britain.* ISDD, London.

8   Parker H, Measham F and Aldridge J (1995) Drug futures: changing patterns of drug use among English youth. *Research Monograph.* **7.** ISDD, London.

9   Health Education Authority (1996) *Drug Realities.* Health Education Authority, London.

10   Greater Glasgow Health Board (1994) *Health Related Behaviour of Young People in Secondary Schools in Glasgow.* Greater Glasgow Health Board, Glasgow.

11   McC Miller P and Plant M (1996) Drinking, smoking and illicit drug use among 15 and 16 year olds in the United Kingdom. *BMJ.* **313:** 394–7.

12   Ramsey M and Piercey A (1996) *Drug Misuse Declared: results of the 1994 British Crime Survey.* Home Office, London.

13   Anon (1996) *Drug Abuse Briefing.* Institute for the Study of Drug Dependence, London.

14   Young J (1971) *The Drugtakers – The Social Meaning of Drug Use.* Paladin, London.

15   NHS Health Advisory Service (1996) *Children and Young People: substance misuse services.* HMSO, London.

16   Coggans N, Sherwan D, Henderson M *et al.* (1991) *National Evaluation of Drug Education in Scotland.* ISDD, London.

17   Dorn N and Murji K (1992) *Drug Prevention: a review of the English language literature.* ISDD, London.

18   Cohen J (1996) Drug education: politics, propaganda and censorship. *Drug Link.* March/April, 12–14. ISDD, London.

19   Greenwood J (1992) Unpopular patients: GPs' attitudes to drug users. *Drug Link.* July/August, 8–10. ISDD, London.

Chapter 12

1   Department of Health (1991) *Drug Misuse and Dependence: Guidelines on Clinical Management.* HMSO, London.

2   Advisory Council on the Misuse of Drugs (1993) *AIDS and Drug Misuse Update.* Department of Health, London.

Chapter 13

1   Report of an Independent Review of Drug Treatment Services in England (1996) *The Task Force to Review Services for Drug Misusers.* Department of Health, London.

2   Strang J, Smith M and Spurrell S (1992) The Community Drug Team. *British Journal of Addiction.* **87**: 169–78.

3   Department of Health (1995) *Reviewing shared care arrangements for drug misusers. EL(95)114. Annex A.* Department of Health Circular, London.

4   The Royal College of General Practitioners (1995) *Managing Drug Users in General Practice. Why? How?* Report of a conference organised by the HIV/AIDS working party. RCGP, London.

5   Elander J, Porter S and Hodson S (1994) What role for general practitioners in the care of opiate users? *Addiction Research.* **1**(4): 309–22.

6   Strang J (1984) Abstinence or abundance – what goal? *BMJ.* **289**: 604.

7   Onion C and Janikiewicz S (1993) Heroin users on a methadone programme. Letter. *British Journal of General Practice.* **43**(370): 216–17.

8   Bennett T and Wright R (1986) Opioid users' attitudes towards and use of NHS clinics, general practitioners and private doctors. *British Journal of Addiction.* **81**: 757–63.

9   Cooke C (1995) *Residential Rehabilitation*. A report prepared for the Task Force.

10   Strang J (1994) Drug Abuse. In *Health Care Needs Assessment: the epidemiologically based needs assessment reviews* (A Stevens and J Raftery eds). Radcliffe Medical Press, Oxford. Chapter 18.

11   Preston A and Malinowski A (1993) *The Rehab Handbook: a user's guide to choosing and using residential services for people with drug or alcohol problems*. Distributed by ISDD, London.

12   Maden A, Swinton M and Gunn J (1991) Drug dependence in prisoners. *BMJ*. **302**: 880–1.

13   Inner London Probation Service (1995) Written Evidence presented to the Task Force.

14   Seivewright NA and Donmall M (1995) *National Cocaine Treatment Study*. A report prepared for the Task Force.

15   Durand M, Andrew T and Gossop M (1995) *Drug Misuse: The Forgotten Families*. A Report to the Esmee Fairbairn Charitable Trust. National Addiction Centre, London.

16   *Tackling Drugs Together*. A consultation document on a strategy for England 1995–98. Cm 2678, October 1994. HMSO, London.

Index